THE
BEAUTY
DETOX
DIET

DELICIOUS RECIPES AND FOODS TO LOOK BEAUTIFUL, LOSE WEIGHT, AND FEEL GREAT

Rockridge Press

ISBN: Print 978-1-62315-199-7 | eBook 978-1-62315-200-0

CONTENTS

INTRODUCTION

Do you often feel fatigued or sluggish? Do you suffer from allergies or red, irritated skin? Is your hair thin or dry, your nails cracked, and your skin rough?

If you answered yes to any of these questions, your body may be in dire need of a detox.

Most dictionaries defines the word "detoxification" or "detox" as the removal "of a harmful substance (such as a poison or toxin) or the effect of such" (*Merriam-Webster Online*). You may be familiar with the term "detox" as it applies to drug and alcohol addictions; however, it has another more ubiquitous application. In the modern health and fitness world, the word has become synonymous with "cleanse"—the act of following a particular diet or engaging in certain eating habits to rid the body of accumulated toxins.

Toxins enter your body through a variety of means. Your body absorbs toxins from the air you breathe, the water you drink, the food you eat, the medications you take, and the environments you inhabit. Each and every day your body is exposed to countless toxins that build up in your body over time, hampering the body's healthy function and affecting your appearance. This accumulation of toxins has been linked to skin problems, hormonal disturbances, weight gain, and even increased risk for serious diseases, including cancer.

By changing the way you eat and by managing the substances you expose your body to, you can cleanse yourself of accumulated toxins. Detox diets are becoming increasingly popular as a means of promoting healthful weight loss, but they provide other significant health benefits as well. By detoxifying, you can boost your metabolism and improve the way you function. Cleansing will also improve the health of your skin, hair, and nails, and it may also decrease your risk of developing reproductive disorders and chronic diseases.

In this book, you will learn how toxins enter your body and how following a detox diet can drastically improve your health and appearance. You will also find a collection of healthful, beautifying recipes, as well as a chapter about how movement, massage, and even breathing exercises can detoxify your body. Once you've finished this book, you will be well equipped and ready to start your own detox.

PART 1

Beauty from the Inside Out

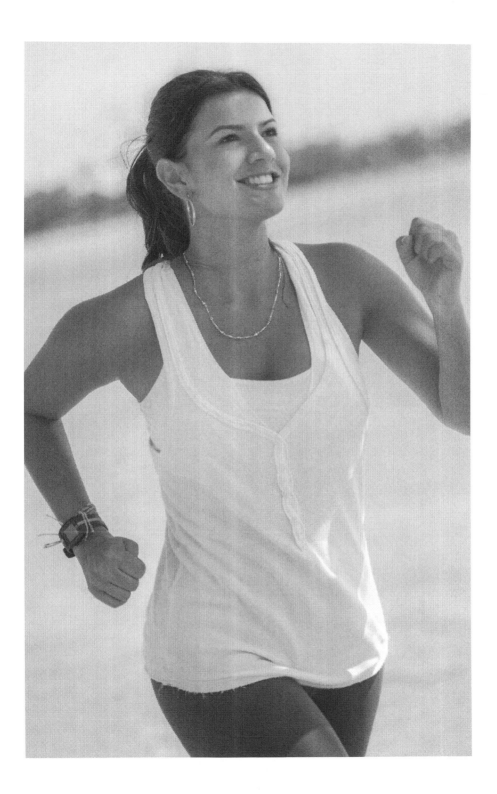

1

IDENTIFYING TOXINS

A toxin is a harmful substance that, even in small doses, can cause serious health problems. When your body is functioning at its highest level, your liver, kidneys, and immune system collaborate to remove toxins as they enter your body. If the intake of toxins exceeds the capacity of your body to handle them, however, the toxins will accumulate until your body can deal with them. It is possible for your body to store toxins for years, and eventually the burden of doing so will become too great, and you will begin to feel the negative effects. As the toxins continue to accumulate, if you do not detox, your body may shut down.

There are a number of different types of toxins, some that are natural, and others that are chemically manufactured. Toxins with a biological origin are called "biotoxins," and they serve two primary purposes: predation and defense. Predators such as snakes, scorpions, spiders, and wasps produce venom that often contains some kind of hemotoxin, necrotoxin, or neurotoxin. Hemotoxins destroy blood cells, while necrotoxins destroy tissues of all types, including skin and muscle tissue. Neurotoxins affect the nervous system. Other types of biotoxins include cyanotoxins (produced by cyanobacteria), apitoxin (produced by honey bees), mycotoxins (produced by fungi), and cytotoxins such as ricin, which attack at the cellular level.

> ## The Beauty | Detox Diet
>
> Almost every time we step outside, put something in our mouth, or apply something to our skin, we are exposing our bodies to toxins. Toxins are present in the air we breathe, the food we eat, and even the environment around us.

The word "toxin" can also be applied to a number of man-made chemicals and compounds. Chemical agents such as herbicides, pesticides, insecticides, and fungicides contain toxic substances, as do many cleaning products, preservatives, detergents, and paints. You may be shocked to hear that the food you eat is also likely to contain either natural or man-made toxins.

Some of the most dangerous toxins that have been found in food are completely natural. Botulinum, for example, is naturally produced by bacteria, and it is one of the most toxic substances known. Dioxin, however, is completely man-made, and it is sixty thousand times more lethal than cyanide. This toxin contaminates crops, which are then fed to cows and other livestock, and it is then passed to us when we ingest meat and dairy products. Toxins can also be found in synthetic dyes and flavors used in processed foods as well as artificial preservatives. Even the fruits and vegetables you buy in the grocery store may be treated with preservatives to prevent spoiling or artificial color to enhance appearance.

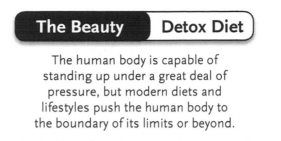

The human body is capable of
standing up under a great deal of
pressure, but modern diets and
lifestyles push the human body to
the boundary of its limits or beyond.

How Does Your Body Become Toxic?

Almost every time we step outside, put something in our mouth,
or apply something to our skin, we are exposing our bodies to toxins. Luckily, our bodies are designed to protect us from harm and
are capable of withstanding a great deal of abuse. Take your skin,
for example: it protects your organs and bones from exposure to
harmful substances. Meanwhile, the immune system is designed
to attack foreign substances that get past the skin. Your digestive
system serves to absorb nutrients and filter out unneeded materials.
Some of the ways you may be exposed to toxins include:

Toxins	Their Sources
LIFESTYLE TOXINS	Addictive substances (drugs, alcohol, etc.)
	Artificial additives, flavors, and preservatives
	Hormone- and antibiotic-treated foods
	Lack of proper sleep and exercise
	Nutritionally deficient diet
	Prescription drugs
	Processed foods
	Refined flours and sugars
ENVIRONMENTAL TOXINS	Air pollution
	Cleaning products
	Heavy metals
	Mold and fungus
	Pesticides and herbicides
	Phthalates (found in plastic)
	Treated/contaminated water
INTERNAL TOXINS	Excess hormones
	Overgrowth of intestinal flora
	Products of metabolic processes
	Repeated cycles of stress
	Suppressing or ignoring emotions

The human body is capable of standing up under a great deal of pressure, but many modern diets and lifestyles push the human body to the boundary of its limits or beyond. When your body becomes overloaded with toxins, your digestive system may fail to function properly, and you may experience numerous problems, including fatigue, muscle aches, bloating, rashes, eczema, acne, water retention, and more. The only way to restore proper bodily function and to reverse these negative effects is to do a "house" cleaning and detox your body.

Exploring Common Toxins in Detail

In the earlier table, you learned some of the many ways toxins are introduced into your body on a daily basis. You probably already understand that overconsumption of addictive substances, abuse of prescription medications, and exposure to chemicals are bad for you, but what about the others on the list? Many people do not realize just how dangerous processed foods and other everyday toxins are. The information you learn in this section may shock you and make you think twice before putting that box of snack cakes in your cart on your next trip to the grocery store.

Lifestyle Toxins

Artificial Coloring—Many Americans shop with their stomachs, and they are more likely to purchase something if it looks good. The food industry has learned to capitalize on this by utilizing thousands of coloring agents to alter and improve the appearance of food. Many of these coloring agents are synthetic, derived from coal tar, and some have even been banned because they are thought to cause cancer. Artificial coloring is commonly used in beverages, candy, canned foods, and even fruits and eggs.

Artificial Flavoring—Flavorings are the most common type of food additive, and they can be either natural or artificial. The food industry uses more than two thousand different flavorings, many of which are made of chemicals. One of the most common artificial flavorings is MSG (monosodium glutamate), which has been known to cause allergic reactions, headaches, chest pains, depression, and other behavioral reactions. The FDA recognizes these flavorings as generally safe for consumption, so food manufacturers are not required to list the details of these products on labels.

Artificial Sweeteners—In recent years, there has been an increasing demand for "sugar-free" foods. The food industry has obliged with a number of artificial sweeteners, which contain few or no calories while still providing the sweet taste people crave. The bad news is that many of these sweeteners are completely artificial and have been linked to a number of health problems, including hyperactivity, behavioral problems, allergies, and cancer.

Preservatives—These substances are a type of additive that the food industry uses to keep food from spoiling. Some of the most common preservatives used are nitrates and nitrites. These substances have been known to trigger allergic reactions and have also been linked to asthma, nausea, headaches, and vomiting. Preservatives aren't just used in canned and frozen foods, though: sulfur dioxide is a type of preservative often used to treat fresh fruits and vegetables to prevent brown spots. By bleaching out rot, these preservatives make it more difficult to pick out inferior produce, and it also destroys the vitamin B that is naturally contained in the food.

Refined Sugar and Flour—To refine something is to remove impurities or to make improvements. With that definition in mind, you might think that refining sugar and flour is a good thing when, in fact, the exact opposite is true. Refined flour is made by stripping the husk of the grain away from the starch. Without the fiber of the husk, these refined starches are quickly absorbed and broken down by the body into sugar. This causes spikes in blood glucose levels and increases the risk for obesity. Refining food products also results in the loss of many valuable vitamins and minerals—often between 50 and 90 percent of the product's natural content.

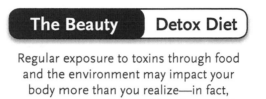

The Beauty Detox Diet

Regular exposure to toxins through food and the environment may impact your body more than you realize—in fact, you may not understand just how much it affects your body until you detox.

Environmental Toxins

Air Pollution—Every year, air pollution is associated with more than one million deaths and innumerable illnesses around the world. Some of the major contributors to air pollution are industrial processes, combustion from automobiles, and airborne pollutants such as pesticides, radioactive fallout, and dust from agricultural practices. Pollution has been linked to increased risk for asthma as well as stunted lung growth, particularly in children.

Household Chemicals—If you were to visit all of the rooms in your house, collecting all the bottles from under sinks, in storage closets, and in your garage, you might be surprised by how much you find. Cleaning products, insect repellents, and even beauty products can contain toxic chemicals. These chemicals are particularly dangerous for children and pets, and they have been linked to cancer, learning disabilities, and reproductive disorders.

Mold—Mold is actually a type of fungus that is often found in damp, humid environments. A wet basement, for example, is a perfect environment for mold. While many mold spores are benign, prolonged exposure or inhalation of large quantities of the spores can lead to respiratory problems. Mold is particularly dangerous for individuals suffering from immunodeficiency disorders.

Phthalates and Heavy Metals—Phthalates are chemical compounds containing phthalic acid, which are found in many types of plastic, including water bottles, food containers, and toys. These substances have been linked to increased risk for birth defects, elevated cancer rates, and other health problems. Heavy metals such as mercury, lead, and arsenic are extremely toxic to the human body—particularly for children. You may be exposed to these metals by consuming fish from contaminated waters, through exposure to lead-based paints, or through mining or smelting activities.

Treated/Contaminated Water—The water you drink potentially contains dozens—even hundreds—of pollutants and chemicals. All of the things you put into your body (prescription drugs, illegal drugs, artificial food additives, etc.) eventually end up in the water supply. Add to that agricultural runoff, illegal waste dumping, and other pollutants, and you are left with water that is not as clean as you think. Cities treat their water with chemicals to remove toxins and impurities, but trace amounts of dangerous substances may still be present. Also, when treating tap water, some of the natural minerals that are good for your body may also be lost.

The Beauty | Detox Diet

Detoxing your body will do more than just improve the way it functions—it will also improve your energy, clear up your skin, improve your sleep habits, and reduce your risk for serious disease.

Internal Toxins

Metabolic Processes—Toxins are a natural by-product of certain metabolic processes, such as breaking down and digesting food. These processes create toxic by-products such as carbon dioxide and ammonia that need to be eliminated from the body. The liver is instrumental in filtering out and excreting toxins, but if the function of the liver is impaired, it could result in the accumulation of toxins.

Overgrowth of Intestinal Flora—Small intestinal bacterial overgrowth (SIBO) is a condition in which the bacteria in the small intestine reproduce too rapidly. In small amounts, these bacteria help to promote healthy digestion, but in large quantities they can cause problems. Certain bacteria produce toxins, which can damage the intestines, causing a number of gastrointestinal problems, such as diarrhea, inflammation, and malabsorption of nutrients.

Stress—Prolonged or repeated cycles of stress can become very toxic to your body. Stress may be induced by emotional trauma, mental illness, a difficult job, and even relationships. Over time, the accumulation of toxic stress can have a negative effect on your physical and mental health. In children, toxic stress has been shown to interrupt healthy brain development, increasing the risk for cognitive impairment.

What Are the Benefits of Detoxing?

Think back to when you ate a particularly large meal or spent a whole weekend eating nothing but fast food, takeout, and pizza. Did you feel bloated or heavy? Was your skin oily or irritated? Perhaps you had difficulty sleeping afterward or had low energy and concentration. While this example may be taken to the extreme, many people do not realize that their bodies are not operating at their full potential.

Regular exposure to toxins through food and environment may impact your body more than you realize—in fact, you may not understand just how much it affects your body until you detox.

It is one thing to say that detoxing your body will help your body function more efficiently, but it's another thing entirely to truly experience it. Chances are, you feel fine right now and are not dealing with any major health problems. If you really think about it, however, you can probably identify several areas where you could stand to see an improvement. Detoxing your body will do more than just improve the way it functions internally—it will also improve your energy, clear up your skin, improve your sleep habits, and reduce your risk for serious disease.

Some of the benefits of detoxing include:

- Balanced hormone levels
- Clearer skin and fewer breakouts
- Improved digestion and regular bowel movements
- Improved quality of sleep
- Increased energy and concentration
- Lowered risk for chronic diseases (e.g., cancer, diabetes, heart disease)
- More stable mood
- Reduced cravings for sugar and junk food
- Reduced stress levels
- Strengthened immune system

Detox Quiz

To find out whether or not your body is in need of a detox, take the time to complete this quiz. After answering the questions, tally up the total number of times you answered "yes" and the number of times you answered "no."

1. Do you often feel sluggish or tired?
   - ☐ Yes
   - ☐ No

2. Do you suffer from allergies (food-related or environmental)?
   - ☐ Yes
   - ☐ No

3. Do you tend to catch colds easily or are you sick often?
   - ☐ Yes
   - ☐ No

4. Do you experience gas, bloating, or indigestion after eating?
   - ☐ Yes
   - ☐ No

5. Do you have dark circles or puffiness under your eyes?
   - ☐ Yes
   - ☐ No

6. Is your skin dry or do you suffer from eczema or psoriasis?
   - ☐ Yes
   - ☐ No

7. Do you have breakouts or other acne problems on a regular basis?
   - ☐ Yes
   - ☐ No

8. Do you have irregular bowel movements?
   - ☐ Yes
   - ☐ No

9. Do you currently, or did you at one point in your life, smoke cigarettes?
   - ☐ Yes
   - ☐ No

10. Do you consume alcoholic beverages more than once a month?
    ☐   Yes
    ☐   No

11. Do you drink an average of fewer than three cups of water per day?
    ☐   Yes
    ☐   No

12. Do you eat fewer than three servings of vegetables per day?
    ☐   Yes
    ☐   No

13. Do you currently take prescription or over-the-counter medications?
    ☐   Yes
    ☐   No

14. Do you use commercial cleaning products and laundry detergent?
    ☐   Yes
    ☐   No

15. Do you wear cosmetics or use commercial hair products?
    ☐   Yes
    ☐   No

16. Do you often experience headaches or fatigue?
    ☐   Yes
    ☐   No

17. Do you experience muscle or joint pain on a regular basis?
    ☐   Yes
    ☐   No

18. Do you wear cologne or perfume?
    ☐   Yes
    ☐   No

19. Do you use pesticides or weed killer on your property?
    ☐ Yes
    ☐ No

20. Do you drink unfiltered tap water?
    ☐ Yes
    ☐ No

1–5: Room for Improvement

If you answered "Yes" to 5 of these questions or fewer, chances are you have already begun to take steps toward detoxifying your body. A detox may still be beneficial, however, to cleanse your body from accumulated toxins.

6–12: Detox Recommended

If you answered "Yes" to between 6 and 12 of these questions, a detox will likely be highly beneficial for you. If you have never done a detox before, this is a great time to start. Cleanse your body of accumulated wastes and toxins and you will feel lighter, more energetic, and healthier than ever before.

13–20: Detox Emergency

If you answered "Yes" to 13 or more of these questions, your body is in dire need of a detox. Based on your answers to these questions, you are putting a significant amount of toxins into your body on a regular basis. If you put too many toxins into your body, it will eventually overpower your body's ability to eliminate them. The toxins will then be stored in your fat cells and organs, contributing to many of the side effects mentioned above.

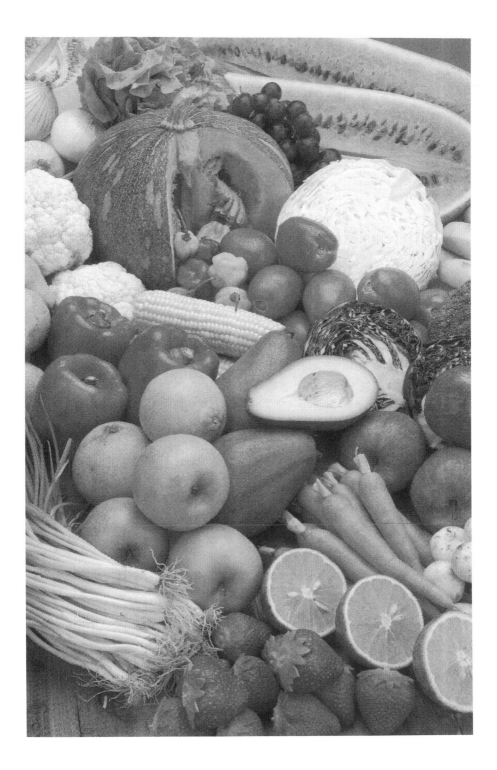

2

HOW TOXINS AFFECT YOU

After reading the first chapter of this book, you should already understand that the buildup of toxins in your body can result in you feeling less than your best. Your digestive system may be sluggish, you might have trouble sleeping, and you could feel bloated or full even when you have not eaten a particularly large meal. Your body is equipped to eliminate the toxins you take in, but if your toxin intake exceeds the ability of your body to handle them, your body might start storing them, which could result in a number of physical side effects.

The first place your body will begin to store toxins is in your fat cells. Your body may also start to store toxins in your ligaments, bones, and even muscle tissue. As more toxins accumulate, you could begin to experience aches or joint pain. If the accumulation continues, it may spread to cellular tissue, resulting in the dysfunction of an organ or the development of a health condition such as impaired vision, heart failure, or pulmonary disease.

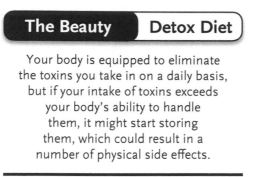

The Beauty · Detox Diet

Your body is equipped to eliminate
the toxins you take in on a daily basis,
but if your intake of toxins exceeds
your body's ability to handle
them, it might start storing
them, which could result in a
number of physical side effects.

In addition to affecting the way you feel physically, toxins can also have an effect on your emotional well-being. A number of toxins, especially environmental ones, have been linked to disturbances and changes in the body's hormonal systems. Toxins have been known to cause numerous mental health problems, including depression and anxiety, by altering or hampering the healthy function of the brain.

Toxins can also affect your brain by altering or inhibiting the activity of neurotransmitters, which are the chemicals in the brain that transmit signals, facilitating communication between your brain and nerve cells. When these neurotransmitters are damaged, it could affect the production of certain chemicals within the brain, such as serotonin, which could affect your mood. In addition, toxins can damage the structure of the brain itself. Neurotoxins such as lead and mercury are known to kill brain cells, affecting behavior, mood, coordination, and even intelligence.

How Toxins Affect the Way You Look

Skin problems can be incredibly embarrassing, especially when they continue to plague you into adulthood. Unfortunately, the modern Western diet does little to repair skin problems. In fact, the food you eat and the toxins you encounter on a daily basis are partially responsible for things like redness, blackheads, inflammation, and pimples. The more toxins present in your body, the more it will affect the way you look. Your skin is the largest organ in your body, and it may also be acting as a storage unit for toxins. When the other detoxifying organs—your liver, kidneys, and lungs—are overloaded with toxins, your skin ends up picking up the slack.

Not only do excess internal toxins end up in your skin, but your skin also absorbs toxins from the environment around you and from the products you put on it. Everything from lotions, shampoos, fragrances, and cosmetics potentially contain toxins that can damage your skin. Toxins from the environment may also enter your skin either by being absorbed through the air or through skin contact with soil or water. All of these toxins block your pores, resulting in acne, greasy skin, and other skin problems.

The Beauty   Detox Diet

Your skin eliminates toxins by pushing them through your pores to the surface of your skin. If too many toxins accumulate in your skin, however, it could lead to redness, inflammation, or breakouts.

Toxins and the Aging Process

Before you can understand how toxins affect the aging process, you need to understand the aging process itself. Many people don't consider themselves to be aging until they hit the thirty- or forty-year mark. In reality, however, you start aging from the moment you are born.

Your body is made up of around one trillion individual cells, and as many as one billion of those cells die every minute that you are alive. These cells do regenerate, but the rate of regeneration versus cell death slows over time. As you get older, the cells in your body will start dying more quickly than they can be regenerated.

Aging is a completely natural process and it cannot be avoided. There are certain factors, however, that speed up the aging process. Nutritional deficiencies and high levels of stress, for example, can accelerate the aging process, making you look and/or feel older than your true age. The buildup of toxins in the body also contributes to accelerated aging by hastening the rate at which cells die without also increasing the rate of regeneration. Keep in mind that, as a whole, your body can handle a significant amount of toxins. The individual cells, on the other hand, can be killed by even the smallest amount, and these cell deaths are *in addition to* the cell deaths that occur naturally.

The human body is designed to efficiently absorb nutrients, filtering out and eliminating waste products and toxins. If you put more toxins in your body than it can handle, however, the excess toxins will be set aside and stored. Extreme toxin buildup can lead to serious diseases, including age-related disorders such as osteoporosis, Alzheimer's, and osteoarthritis. Detoxifying your body will help flush out those excess toxins, restoring your body's natural rhythm and stopping additional cell death.

Detoxing for Healthy Skin and Hair

Earlier in this chapter you learned how toxicity can affect your skin, but you may be curious about just how that process works. Your skin is made up of two primary layers: the epidermis and the dermis (which includes sebaceous glands). The epidermis is the outermost layer of skin from which dead skin cells are shed, taking toxins they contain along with them. The second layer of skin is the dermis, which constantly regenerates, forming new skin cells and pushing old skin cells to the top to be shed. The sebaceous glands secrete sebum, which is an oily matter that lubricates and waterproofs the skin as well as releases toxins from fat cells.

Every day, your body sheds between two and three billion dead cells. In addition to eliminating toxins through the shedding of dead skin cells, toxins and impurities can also be released through sweat glands. Thus, exercising to induce sweating is an easy way to boost your body's natural detoxification. Though your skin does eliminate some of the toxins in your body on a daily basis, many people's bodies are still "toxic" in that they contain more toxins than the body can handle. It is in cases like this where a detox diet can be especially effective.

Before engaging in a detox, it is important to realize that you are likely to experience some side effects. Remember, the goal of detoxifying your body is to eliminate excess toxins, and those toxins have to go somewhere. One of the many ways in which those toxins will be released is through your skin. You shouldn't be surprised, then, if you experience an increase in blemishes or skin oil during the first few days of your detox. Don't worry—once you have cleansed your body of excess toxins, you will see the healthy, glowing skin you've been wanting.

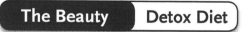

The Beauty Detox Diet

By cleansing your body and skin of toxins, you will be unclogging your pores, which will result in a clearer complexion. Not only can a detox improve the health of your skin, but it may also restore your hair to its natural beauty.

By cleansing your body and skin of toxins, you will be unclogging your pores, which will result in a clearer complexion. You will experience relief from acne, uneven texture, and excess oil. You may also experience a reduction in fine lines, age spots, and dark circles under the eyes as a result of improved capillary circulation. Not only can a detox improve the health of your skin, but it may also improve your hair. After detoxing, you can expect your hair to be smooth, shiny, and soft. Chemical-laced hair products can dry out or damage your hair, making it frizzy and unmanageable. Detoxing can restore your hair to its natural beauty.

Detoxing for Organ Health

One of the main organs involved in eliminating toxins from the body is the liver. It plays an essential role not only in eliminating toxins, but also in breaking down nutrients and producing red blood cells. The liver is largely responsible for detoxifying harmful substances, and it fulfills this role in several ways: by filtering the blood to eliminate toxins; by synthesizing and excreting bile to get rid of fat-soluble vitamins like cholesterol; and by producing enzymes that neutralize harmful chemicals. Your liver acts without regard to where the toxins come from—it treats those produced by your body the same way it treats toxins from food, medications, and environmental factors.

Your lungs, kidneys, and intestines also play a role in removing toxins. The lungs, for example, filter out allergens, mold, and other airborne toxins. Your kidneys are responsible for filtering your blood and diverting waste products to the bladder so they can be eliminated. If any of these organs becomes overworked or bogged down with excess fat, inflammation, or toxin accumulation, it could limit your body's natural detoxification abilities. Detoxifying will help restore proper function to your organs.

Below you will find valuable information regarding your organs' roles in detoxifying the body as well as information on what happens when these organs aren't functioning to full capacity.

Kidneys

Your kidneys are the primary detoxifying organs of your urinary system. They filter your blood, removing wastes and diverting them to the bladder so they can be eliminated from your body. Your kidneys also help regulate mineral levels and electrolytes to prevent toxic buildup.

If the function of your kidneys is impaired, they may not be able to properly filter toxins from your blood. Kidney disease and damage is often caused by high blood pressure, diabetes, poor eating habits, inflammation, and overuse or prolonged exposure to medications and toxic chemicals.

Liver

As has already been mentioned, the liver is the most important organ for detoxification. It breaks down nutrients and toxic substances, excreting toxins through bile and urine.

Unfortunately, liver disease is a fairly common problem and it can affect your liver's ability to properly filter out toxins. Some of the most common causes of liver disease and damage include excessive alcohol intake, poor diet, and abuse of drugs or other toxic chemicals.

Lungs

Your lungs are the first organs to come into contact with airborne toxins, and they serve to filter these toxins and other harmful substances out of the air you breathe. The lungs are also responsible for delivering oxygen to your blood.

Shallow breathing can greatly reduce the efficiency of your lungs in detoxifying the body. This can be caused by or exacerbated by a poor diet, air pollution, and smoking.

Skin

You may be surprised to hear that your skin is responsible for eliminating about one-third of the toxins, bacteria, and viruses that enter your body. If the other detoxifying organs (liver, kidneys, and lungs) become overworked, your skin steps up to take on the extra load.

Your skin eliminates toxins by pushing them through your pores to the surface. If too many toxins accumulate in your skin, however, it could lead to redness, inflammation, or breakouts.

Detoxing for Weight Loss

You probably already know that if you eat more calories than you burn, you will gain weight. You may not know, however, some of the additional factors that play into weight gain and weight loss. Adipose tissue is the type of tissue used by the body to store energy in the form of lipids (fat). This type of tissue is typically found beneath the skin, but in cases where there is too much adipose tissue, it can begin to back up in and around the organs. Your liver, the largest internal organ in your body, is especially prone to storing excess fat. The more fat stored in your liver, the less efficient it will be.

The food you eat and the other toxins you put into your body have a direct effect on the condition of your liver and on your ability to lose weight. In addition to the toxins you put into your body, your liver may also begin to produce its own toxins as it works overtime trying to digest all of the excess sugar, fat, and other components of processed foods. The toxins your liver cannot immediately deal with are stored in fat cells, which leads to weight gain. If your liver is healthy and you eat a diet of clean, wholesome foods, your liver will be able to handle all of the toxins that enter your body, and it will metabolize your fat cells for energy rather than storing them.

Detoxing will provide a number of benefits, but one of the most important ones is that it will clean up your liver. This is an essential step in achieving healthful weight loss, because unless your liver is able to break down the food you eat (eliminating the toxins rather than storing them), you may have difficulty losing weight no matter how hard you try. Detoxing will help you to eliminate stored toxins, cleaning up your internal organs so they can resume their proper functions. In addition to cleansing your body, the detox diet will also help you reorient your eating habits so you are more likely to lose weight and keep it off for good.

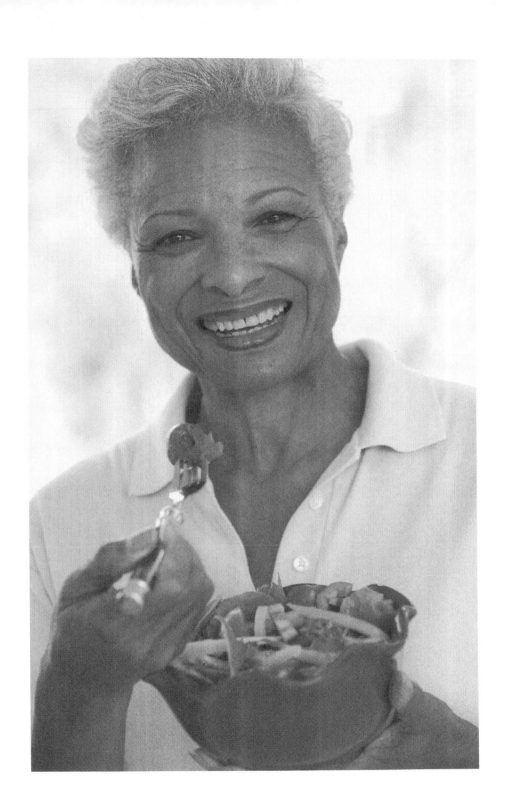

3

THE BEAUTY OF DETOXING

If your body is not able to fully process and absorb nutrients from the food you eat, your detox may not be completely effective. Remember, the goal of a detox is to cleanse your body of toxins and to repair the damage done. In this chapter, we'll look at the role probiotics and enzymes play in this process and discuss whether or not a more thorough internal cleanse might be right for you.

Incorporating Probiotics

Probiotics are bacteria that help promote healthy digestion by encouraging a balance in the microflora of the intestines. Your digestive tract contains almost four hundred different kinds of bacteria that help protect you from harmful bacteria and aid in healthy digestion. The word "probiotic" may also be applied to dietary supplements containing live bacteria taken for the purpose of improving gut health and digestion. These products can be taken to reduce or prevent gas, diarrhea, and bloating. They may also help control the symptoms of inflammatory bowel disease.

Because healthy digestion is such an important component of a detox, probiotics can be a great supplement to your detox diet. In addition, probiotics may help repair damage done to the intestinal tract by poor diet and inflammation or infections. If your body is not able to fully process and absorb nutrients from the food you eat, your detox may not be completely effective. Remember, the goal of a detox is to cleanse your body of toxins and to repair the damage done.

One option for increasing the healthful bacteria in your body is to take probiotic supplements. These often take the form of a daily pill or tablet that delivers the probiotics directly to your digestive system. Another option is to include some naturally probiotic foods into your diet. Some examples of probiotic foods include sauerkraut, kefir (generally considered a good dairy product), and pickles. Incorporating some of these foods into your detox diet will help you boost your body's absorption of key nutrients while also enabling improved digestion and natural detoxification.

The Role of Enzymes

Enzymes are the molecules in the body that are responsible for catalyzing (increasing the chemical reaction rates) of bodily processes. These molecules initiate every action that takes place in or involving the human body. This includes simple actions such as blinking as well as complex processes such as food digestion. In addition, enzymes are instrumental in breaking down and removing dead and damaged cells and tissue. When the enzyme levels in your body drop too low, diseased cells and tissues will accumulate in the body rather than being shed.

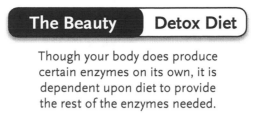

Though your body does produce certain enzymes on its own, it is dependent upon diet to provide the rest of the enzymes needed.

The pancreas is an essential component of the digestive system in that it produces the enzymes needed to break down food and process nutrients. It is responsible for transporting pancreatic enzymes into the duodenum (the first section of the small intestine that is responsible for using the enzymes to break down food), helping to neutralize stomach acid entering your small intestine. There are three types of enzymes produced by the pancreas: lipase, protease, and amylase. A shortage of any of these can result in diarrhea, malabsorption of nutrients, or damage to the intestines due to toxic buildup.

Though your body does produce certain enzymes on its own, it is dependent upon your diet to provide the rest of the enzymes needed. If your diet doesn't provide enough enzymes, not only will it affect your digestion, but it will also decrease your body's natural detoxification. Eating raw foods such as fruits and vegetables is the best way to ensure you get enough enzymes in your diet. Cooking and processing food destroys many of the enzymes contained within it, so eat as many raw foods as you can.

Foods that are high in enzymes include:

- Bean sprouts
- Dried fruit

- Fresh carrot juice
- Fresh tomato juice
- Kefir
- Oysters
- Papaya and papaya seeds
- Pineapple
- Raw almonds
- Salmon roe
- Sauerkraut
- Sprouted seeds

Fasting for Detoxification

Incorporating probiotics and enzymes into your diet will definitely improve the efficacy of your detoxing, but there are still more ways to increase the benefits you receive. Not only is the type of food you eat important for detoxing, but the amount you eat and the frequency of your meals may also be significant. Fasting is a practice that people of most cultures have practiced in one form or another for thousands of years. Recent medical evidence suggests that fasting may not only encourage weight loss, but also boost the results of a detox.

A fast can be defined as the act of abstaining from food, liquid, or both for a defined period of time. A full fast, or absolute fast, is a period of abstinence from both food and liquid. One method of fasting that has recently become popular is intermittent fasting. This involves incorporating one or more nonconsecutive fasting days per week while engaging in normal eating habits on non-fast days. Though there is a great deal of debate regarding the efficacy of fasting for detoxification, a significant amount of scientific research suggests that fasting encourages the body to enter a state of ketosis, a biochemical process that occurs during fat burning. This is the most effective state for the body to be in for the removal of toxins. As you already know, when your body's natural detoxification processes are inhibited, your body begins to store excess toxins in your fat cells. In a state of ketosis, the body begins to burn fat cells for energy, thus releasing stored toxins so they can be eliminated (Foster 1967).

The Beauty | **Detox Diet**

Though there is a great deal of debate regarding the efficacy of fasting for detoxification, a significant amount of scientific research suggests that fasting encourages the body to enter a state of ketosis—the most effective state for the body to be in for toxin removal.

It is important to understand the proper way to engage in fasting for detoxification. Abstaining from all food and liquid for an extended period of time can be extremely dangerous. The best way to engage in a fast to boost your body's detoxification is to incorporate twenty-four-hour fasts on a weekly, bimonthly, or monthly basis. While engaging in a fast, it is essential that you provide your body with plenty of water along with some form of nutrition. Fresh fruit and vegetable juices are great options for fasts because they will provide your body with healthful nutrients while also boosting the effects of your detox. If you plan to engage in a fast lasting more than two to three days, consult your doctor first.

Colonics and Enemas

In researching natural detox methods, you may come across information regarding colonics and enemas. Both of these services are designed to cleanse the colon by encouraging it to expel its contents. Over time and through unhealthful diets, the colon can become clogged with old fecal matter, resulting in accumulation of harmful bacteria, distension of the colon, and a variety of other diseases or side effects, including constipation, hemorrhoids, irritable bowel syndrome, Crohn's disease, and colon/rectal cancer. There are a number of ways to clean out the colon including a colonic, an enema, or a colon detox.

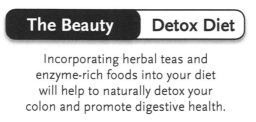

The Beauty | Detox Diet

Incorporating herbal teas and
enzyme-rich foods into your diet
will help to naturally detox your
colon and promote digestive health.

An enema is a procedure which introduces liquid into the colon and rectum through the anus. This results in the expansion and evacuation of the lower intestinal tract. Enemas can be administered at home, and they are often preferred as a method of colon cleansing because of how fast they work. A colonic, also called colon hydrotherapy, is a similar procedure in that water is injected into the colon through the rectum. The main difference is that this procedure requires the use of special equipment. Colonic machines also have the capacity to administer an amount of water equivalent to six or seven enemas within one hour.

Some medical professionals suggest that regular use of enemas and other colon cleansing procedures may not only be unnecessary but also harmful. Improper administration of enemas can result in a loss of colon muscle tone, which may eventually prevent normal bowel movement. And colonics have actually been made illegal in some states by the American Medical Association (AMA); in other areas, it may be difficult to find a trained technician. A safer, healthier alternative to either of these procedures is a natural colon detox. Incorporating herbal teas and enzyme-rich foods into your diet will help to naturally detox your colon and promote digestive health.

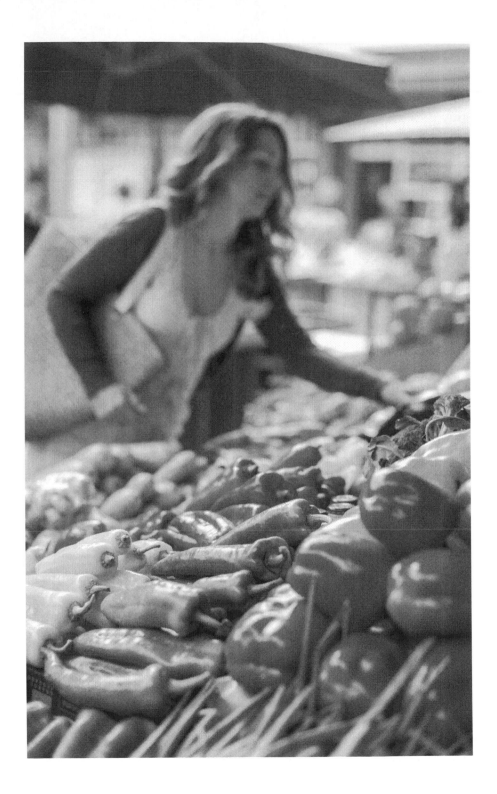

4

A BEAUTIFUL PANTRY—
WHAT TO KEEP, WHAT TO DISCARD

You have probably heard the saying "you are what you eat," but you may not realize just how applicable that statement is. While eating a fast-food hamburger may not cause you to turn into a hamburger, the toxins and other unhealthful ingredients contained in the burger will have an effect on your body. The more unhealthful foods you eat, the more toxic your body will become. Over time, the symptoms of toxicity will compound, and you will feel increasingly sick and tired. Rather than hounding your doctor for prescription medications, turn to the only solution that truly works—detoxifying your body by eating whole, nutritious foods.

This detox diet isn't about following a certain meal plan or eating a certain number of calories. It is about eliminating foods that introduce toxins into your body and replacing them with naturally detoxifying foods. In this chapter, you will find a list of food categories to include in your detox diet as well as a list of foods to avoid. Completely eliminating processed foods can be a challenge for some people, especially for those whose diet is almost entirely composed of these foods. To get the best results from your detox, however, it is important that you stick to the guidelines of the diet as closely as possible.

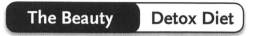

The Beauty | **Detox Diet**

Rather than hounding your doctor
for prescription medications,
turn to the only solution that truly
works—detoxifying your body by
eating whole, nutritious foods.

Healthful foods to include in your detox:

- Dairy substitutes
- Fresh fruits
- Fresh herbs and spices
- Gluten-free grains
- Green vegetables
- Lean animal protein
- Natural beverages
- Natural sweeteners
- Non-vegetable oils
- Nuts and seeds
- Vegetable proteins

Fresh Fruits

Not only are fresh fruits an important element in a detox diet, they are also delicious. Fruits are naturally packed with healthful vitamins and minerals to give your body the nutrition it needs. Additionally, fruits help reduce excess toxicity by eliminating acidic chemicals and balancing your body's pH. Fruits also encourage your body to utilize all of its detoxification methods—your body will become more efficient in eliminating waste. Other benefits include increased energy and improvements in cognitive function, eyesight, skin health, and hair condition.

Good detox fruits include:

- Apples
- Blueberries
- Cherries
- Cranberries

- Figs
- Grapes
- Grapefruit
- Kiwis

- Lemons
- Limes
- Oranges
- Strawberries

The Beauty   Detox Diet

Incorporating fresh fruits into your diet will help your body utilize all of its detoxification methods— your body will become more efficient in eliminating waste.

Green Vegetables

Green vegetables are an essential ingredient in a detox diet because they provide your body with a wealth of vital nutrients. Many vegetables such as asparagus are high in antioxidants and natural probiotics, which help stimulate the growth of good bacteria in the gut. Other vegetables such as artichokes contain high levels of cynarin, a natural chemical that increases bile production and liver function to help flush toxins out of your system.

Vegetables can be consumed raw, cooked, or in juice form. Feel free to add some fresh fruit to your juicing recipes to enhance the flavor.

Good vegetables for detox include:

- Artichokes
- Arugula
- Asparagus
- Beets
- Broccoli
- Brussels Sprouts
- Cabbage
- Carrots
- Cauliflower
- Collard Greens
- Cucumbers
- Dandelion Greens
- Kale
- Lettuce
- Onions

Fresh Herbs and Spices

Not only are fresh herbs and spices a great way to add flavor to your favorite dishes, they can also boost your detox diet. Turmeric, which can also be found in dried form, is especially beneficial for the liver—it helps boost bile production to flush toxins from the body. Cilantro binds specifically to heavy metals like mercury and lead, making it easier for your body to eliminate them. Garlic performs a similar role in addition to strengthening the immune system. Many herbs and spices, such as ginger, are useful in restoring healthy digestion—this is essential for detoxing because toxins often cause damage to the digestive system.

Good herbs and spices for detox include:

- Basil
- Cilantro
- Cinnamon
- Dill
- Fennel
- Garlic
- Ginger
- Lemongrass
- Mint
- Parsley
- Peppermint
- Turmeric

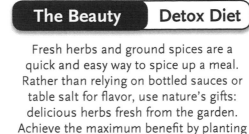

The Beauty **Detox Diet**

Fresh herbs and ground spices are a
quick and easy way to spice up a meal.
Rather than relying on bottled sauces or
table salt for flavor, use nature's gifts:
delicious herbs fresh from the garden.
Achieve the maximum benefit by planting
an herb garden in your backyard.

Nuts and Seeds

Nuts and seeds are an important part of any healthful diet because
they contain a variety of important nutrients, including protein,
antioxidants, and healthful fats. Brazil nuts, in particular, are great
for detoxing because they are high in selenium, a mineral that helps
boost your white blood cell count. (White blood cells help to fight
off infection.) Another great food to include in your detox diet is
flaxseed. A two-tablespoon serving of flaxseed is enough to satisfy
your recommended daily allowance of omega-3 fatty acids. These
seeds are also loaded with fiber, which helps promote healthful
digestion and the natural elimination of toxins.

Good nuts and seeds for detox include:

- Almonds
- Cashews
- Chestnuts
- Flaxseeds
- Hazelnuts
- Pecans
- Pine Nuts
- Pistachios
- Pumpkin Seeds
- Sesame Seeds
- Sunflower Seeds
- Walnuts

Dairy Substitutes

There are a number of health problems associated with dairy
products (as you will find in the next section). As part of your

detox diet, you should plan to eliminate all dairy products. This doesn't necessarily mean giving up milk—you may just need to switch to a non-dairy variety, such as almond, coconut, or rice milk. These milks are available in lots of different flavors, so you can choose the one you prefer. Avoid using soy milk because soy products are unhealthful.

Natural Sweeteners

Artificial sweeteners are man-made and full of synthetic substances and chemicals that are harmful for your health. As part of your detox diet, plan to utilize natural sweeteners like those listed below. Avoid refined sugars, including white sugar, brown sugar, and cane sugar as well as artificial sweeteners.

Good natural sweeteners for detox include:

- Agave Nectar
- Blackstrap Molasses
- Brown Rice Syrup
- Fruit Sweetener
- Honey
- Stevia

Non-Vegetable Oils

In the next section, you will learn about the dangers of vegetable oils. Many of these oils are derived from genetically altered crops or pressed using chemical processes. As part of your detox diet, plan to incorporate non-vegetable oils such as olive, coconut, and seed oils as an alternative to unhealthful vegetable oils. Olive oil helps boost the immune system and may also reduce your risk for serious diseases like cancer and diabetes. Nut oils are a good source of phytonutrients and also contain high levels of essential vitamins and minerals, like selenium, calcium, and vitamin B complex.

Good non-vegetable oils for detox include:

- Almond
- Coconut
- Flaxseed
- Olive
- Safflower
- Sesame
- Sunflower
- Walnut

Lean Animal Protein

Protein is an essential part of any healthful diet, but you need to be careful what protein sources you choose. In the next section, you will learn about the hidden toxins in dark and processed meats. Lean animal protein from certain types of fish, chicken, turkey, and wild game, however, can be beneficial for a detox diet. These are low in calories but high in protein and other nutrients.

Vegetable Proteins

Aside from lean meats, there are several additional sources of healthful protein you can include in your detox diet. Some of the best sources for vegetable protein include lentils, peas, and beans. Lentils are an excellent source of dietary fiber, iron, and essential amino acids like lysine and isoleucine. Beans such as black beans and kidney beans are slightly lower in protein than lentils, but they still contain a variety of nutrients. The key to eating legumes is to cook them thoroughly to make them more easily digestible.

Gluten-Free Grains

In the next section, you will learn about the dangers of gluten and how it can be found in a majority of prepared breads, pastas, and baked goods. As part of your detox diet, you will need to eliminate these grains, replacing them with gluten-free grains. Certain gluten-free grains are an excellent source of protein and dietary fiber. Being gluten-free, these grains may also relieve digestive stress, which will help you digest your food more appropriately.

Good gluten-free grains for detox include:

- Amaranth
- Brown Rice
- Buckwheat
- Millet
- Oats
- Quinoa
- Red Rice
- Sorghum
- Teff

Natural Beverages

The best beverages for you to drink during your detox include water, decaffeinated herbal tea, seltzer, and mineral water. Water is an essential part of a detox diet because it helps flush toxins from your body. Additionally, water helps keep your brain and body hydrated so they can function properly. Herbal teas are another great option if you prefer a beverage with a little flavor. Ginger, lemon, and herbal teas are especially effective as part of a detox diet. Try making your own combination using loose tea leaves, or buy organic tea bags from your local health food store.

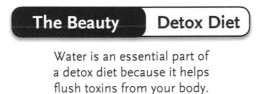

The Beauty   Detox Diet

Water is an essential part of a detox diet because it helps flush toxins from your body.

Toxic Foods to Avoid:

- Alcohol and Soft Drinks
- Artificial Sweeteners
- Dairy Products
- Dark Meats and Fish
- Gluten-Free Grains
- Peanuts and Peanut Butter
- Processed Oils and Dressings
- Soybeans and Soy Products

Dairy Products

You were probably raised with the knowledge that drinking milk will help your bones grow strong. Recent studies suggest, however, that consumption of dairy products might not impact bone growth—in fact, it could be bad for you. A study conducted by Cornell University reveals that the United States is one of the world's largest consumers of dairy products. Strangely, the United States also has some of the highest fracture rates and instances of osteoporosis. The conclusion of this study suggests that there is little evidence to support the idea that increased intake of dairy products promotes bone growth (Lanou, Berkow, and Barnard 2005).

If you think about it, humans are the only species that continue to drink milk after infancy. We are also the only species to drink the milk of another animal. In order to make milk safe for human consumption, it is often pasteurized. While this process kills bacteria and other harmful pathogens, it actually alters the calcium content in milk. Because your body cannot recognize calcium in this altered form, it may be treated as a toxin. Another toxic property of dairy milk is that it contains galactose, a simple sugar broken down from the milk sugar lactose. Galactose has been linked to ovarian cancer and it can also inhibit healthful immune function.

| The Beauty | Detox Diet |

If you think about it, humans are the only species that continue to drink milk after infancy. We are also the only species to drink the milk of another animal.

Dark Meats and Fish

A study conducted by the National Cancer Institute in 2009 and published in the *Archives of Internal Medicine* explores the effects of meat intake on mortality (Sinha et al. 2009). Fatty cuts of meat from pork, beef, and veal contain several different toxins that can damage your health. HNE, or 4-Hydroxynonenal, is a derivative of omega-6 fats. Small amounts of this substance are good for your body, but excess consumption has been linked to chronic diseases such as diabetes and cancer as well as inflammation and cognitive decline. Acrolein is a highly volatile toxin that is produced when the fats in certain types of meat and protein are heated. This toxin is a potent carcinogen, and it has the potential to damage your mitochondrial DNA. Another toxin resulting from cooked fats and protein is glyoxal. Also a carcinogen, glyoxal interrupts cellular signaling in the body.

In addition to fresh cuts of meat, processed and canned meats are also likely to contain toxins. Sodium nitrate is a commonly used preservative in meats and meat products. This preservative helps enhance the color of meat and also extends its shelf life. This artificial additive, however, has been linked to the formation of cancer-causing nitrosamines in the body. Some of the foods most likely to have been treated with sodium nitrate include hot dogs, bacon, sausage, and other packaged meats.

You have probably been told that fish is good for you because it is high in protein and it contains omega-3 fatty acids. While these things are true, certain types of fish are more likely than others to be exposed to methyl mercury, which is incredibly toxic to the human body. Exposure to this toxin has been linked to neurological damage, hearing defects, memory loss, and death. Some of the fish most likely to contain higher levels of methyl mercury include halibut, mackerel, marlin, swordfish, shark, and bluefin tuna. Types of fish having the lowest levels of mercury include salmon, flounder, haddock, and tilapia. Some other seafood also contains low levels of mercury. These include shrimp, crab, oysters, and scallops.

Grains

One of the biggest trends in modern health and fitness cultures is a movement toward eating whole grains. Whole-wheat breads, pastas, and cereals are becoming more and more popular. Claims that whole grains are healthful can be very misleading, especially since many of the foods that are labeled "whole grain" are not made entirely from whole grains. In fact, many so-called whole-grain products are actually worse for you than traditional products. But what makes grains bad for you?

Grains have an addictive quality due to certain peptides they contain called opioids. These substances cause the human body to produce exorphins, which serve to increase your appetite and cause food cravings. In addition to these opioids, grains also contain toxic anti-nutrients such as lectins, gluten, and phytates. Lectins are carbohydrate-binding proteins that can be very toxic to the human body if consumed in excess or not properly cooked. A study published in the *Pakistan Journal of Nutrition* in 2009 revealed that overconsumption of lectins contributes to allergic reactions, gastrointestinal stress, and nutritional deficiencies as well as increased risk for chronic diseases, including celiac disease, diabetes, and cardiovascular disease. The results of the study suggest that lectins also "serve as a vehicle allowing foreign proteins to invade our natural gut defenses and cause damage well beyond the gut" (Hamid and Masood 2009).

Gluten is a type of protein found in wheat, barley, and rye. It has been linked to a number of health problems, primarily food allergies and autoimmune disorders like celiac disease. Dr. Murray (1999) of the Mayo Clinic conducted a study regarding the increased frequency in diagnosing celiac cases since the 1950s. After testing blood samples preserved from the 1950s, Murray found that modern rates for celiac disease were more than four times higher than the preserved blood tested. Based on the results of his study, Murray suggested that the increase may be linked to escalated consumption of grains and grain-based food products. Avoiding gluten-containing grains is the key to reducing food allergies and other gastrointestinal issues.

Soybeans and Soy Products

Soy and soy products have become a staple in the diet of vegetarians and vegans around the world. Soybeans are considered by many to be one of the healthiest foods in the world due to their low-fat, high-quality protein. In reality, however, soy can be very toxic for your body. Not only can it increase your cancer risk, but it may also contribute to infertility in women. Soy contains a number of harmful substances, including goitrogens, lectins, phytates, and protease inhibitors. It can also interfere with estrogen levels, which can have very serious effects for both men and women.

Goitrogens are a type of compound that suppresses the healthful function of the thyroid gland. These compounds interfere with the uptake of iodine, which may result in the enlargement of the thyroid gland. This contributes to hypothyroidism and other thyroid problems, which can result in a decreased metabolism, low energy, and a weakened immune system. Phytates, which are found in both grains and soy, are also very harmful. They bind to certain minerals, such as calcium, iron, magnesium, and zinc, which makes your body unable to absorb those nutrients.

One of the most serious problems caused by soy is its interference with estrogen levels. Men and women both have certain levels of estrogen and testosterone. In men, testosterone levels are higher, and in women, estrogen levels are higher. Soy products contain plant estrogens called isoflavones, which raise the estrogen levels while lowering testosterone. In men, this can lead to decreased libido, loss of energy or stamina, and fat accumulation. In women, high estrogen levels may increase the risk for breast cancer and could impact fertility. Overconsumption of soy can also be very harmful for newborns, because a baby needs to have the proper ratio of hormones in order to develop correctly.

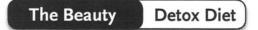

The Beauty   Detox Diet

One of the most serious problems caused by the consumption of soy is its interference with estrogen levels. High estrogen levels may increase the risk for breast cancer and could impact your fertility.

Peanuts and Peanut Butter

Many Americans were raised on peanut butter and jelly sandwiches as well as peanut-flavored candies, ice creams, and other treats. Unfortunately, peanuts and peanut butter are actually quite toxic. Peanuts, despite their name, are actually a legume and are one of the top eight food allergens identified by the United States Food and Drug Administration (FDA). Additionally, peanuts contain lectins, which you have already learned about. What you may not know, however, is that peanuts are highly susceptible to a type of mold that produces a mycotoxin called aflatoxin, which is one of the most carcinogenic substances known to man. A government office in Kenya (where aflatoxin contamination is extreme) published an extensive report on the dangers of aflatoxin in 2011. According to this report, exposure to this toxin often results in altered digestion, improper metabolism of nutrients, edema, and eventual hepatic failure. In children, aflatoxin exposure can also result in delayed development and stunted growth. Though you are unlikely to ingest a toxic dose of aflatoxin with just a handful of peanuts, prolonged exposure to peanuts, peanut butter, and peanut oil can be harmful.

Processed Oils and Dressings

Processed, refined, and hydrogenated oils are a fairly new addition to the modern Western diet. Before the early 1900s, the technology didn't exist to extract oils from certain nuts and seeds. Thanks to new technologies, however, you can now have your choice of a variety of vegetable oils such as canola, soybean, and corn, and butter substitutes like margarine. Olive oil has been around for centuries because it can be made simply by pressing olives. Vegetable oils, on the other hand, require chemical processing and alteration. These oils can be found in a majority of processed foods, and they are also used in salad dressings, marinades, and sauces.

Canola oil, one of the most popular vegetable oils (marketed as low in saturated fats and cholesterol-free), is derived from hybridized rape seeds. Rape plants produce an oil that contains up to 50 percent erucic acid, an incredibly toxic substance. This acid has been linked to a variety of harmful effects in laboratory animals. Additionally, the rape plants from which the oil is derived are genetically modified and treated heavily with pesticides. All vegetable oils contain high levels of polyunsaturated fats, which are easily oxidized by the body. This results in inflammation and cellular mutation. These effects have been linked to reproductive disorders and problems in babies and children.

Artificial Sweeteners

Many food manufacturers have begun utilizing artificial sweeteners in their recipes so they can label their products "sugar-free." Some of the most commonly used artificial sweeteners are aspartame, saccharin, and sucralose. Sugar alcohols such as maltitol and sorbitol are also popular. The benefit of artificial sweeteners is that they are calorie-free. Though many artificial sweeteners have been approved by the FDA, there have been studies linking them to numerous health problems.

A study conducted by the American Society of Nephrology in San Diego recently linked artificial sweeteners to reduced kidney function. Adult women participating in the study who consumed at least two diet sodas per day experienced a 30 percent decrease in kidney function over ten years. Some artificial sweeteners, like sucralose, contain ingredients that have been positively identified as toxic. Overconsumption of artificial sweeteners has also been linked to increased risk for diabetes and metabolic disorders (Lin and Curhan 2011).

Alcohol, Soft Drinks, and Caffeine

There is a reason why people under the influence of alcohol are said to be "intoxicated." Alcohol consumption can be very damaging to the human body. In fact, the word "intoxication" comes from the Latin word for "to poison." Alcohol attaches to the membranes of your nerve cells, affecting their function. This leads to slurred speech, decreased motor function, and impaired judgment. Alcoholics and heavy drinkers often experience serious and permanent effects, such as weakness in the limbs, nerve damage, organ failure, and cancer.

Carbonated beverages and other soft drinks are often sweetened with artificial sweeteners—this is especially common in diet sodas. You have already learned the dangers of artificial sweeteners, but soft drinks contain a number of other toxic ingredients as well. BPA, or bisphenol A, is a type of chemical used to line soda cans. This chemical has been linked to birth defects and improper development in children. Another substance found in soft drinks is phosphoric acid. This chemical interferes with the body's absorption of calcium, which can lean to osteoporosis. It may also neutralize stomach acid, which can result in digestive problems.

Another harmful ingredient found in soft drinks and other popular beverages is caffeine. Caffeine may help keep you awake, but it can also have a devastating effect on your health. This substance has been linked to birth defects, insomnia, high blood pressure, cardiovascular disease, and high cholesterol. Additionally, caffeine is a highly addictive substance, and the effects of withdrawal can be very unpleasant.

The Beauty Detox Diet

Caffeine may help keep you awake, but it can also have a negative effect on your health.

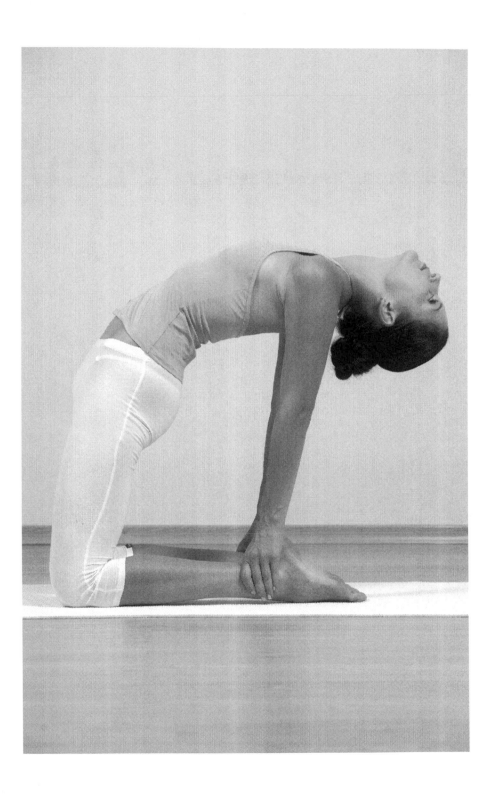

5

BEAUTY AND MOVEMENT

To gain the detox benefits of exercise, you don't need to run a 5K three times a week. Even the simplest forms of exercise stimulate an increase in blood flow throughout your body. There are many ways to move your body, and all of them help in the detoxification process.

Detox Benefits of Exercise

One of the side effects of toxin accumulation is that you may begin to feel sluggish or low in energy. As a result, you may find yourself exercising less often, which will only exacerbate the problem. Exercise is actually a very efficient method of detoxification for a number of reasons. Primarily, it causes your body to sweat, which eliminates toxins from your body through your pores. Exercising may also cause you to breathe more deeply, allowing more oxygen into your lungs so it can be carried by your blood throughout the body.

With increased blood flow, your organs begin to work more efficiently, which enhances the detox process. With increased blood circulation comes increased circulation of lymph fluids, which help remove toxins and other harmful substances. An added benefit of exercise is that it helps you to lose weight by burning fat cells, where toxins are often stored.

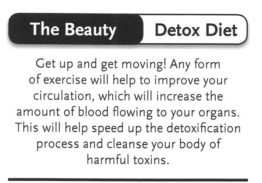

The Beauty **Detox Diet**

Get up and get moving! Any form of exercise will help to improve your circulation, which will increase the amount of blood flowing to your organs. This will help speed up the detoxification process and cleanse your body of harmful toxins.

If you are not used to getting regular exercise, it is a good idea to start off slow and build up as you increase your endurance. Start with a fifteen-minute walk three times a week, eventually building toward a daily walk of the same length (or longer). You can also try shorter periods of jogging at a moderate pace or riding a bike, if you prefer. Another exercise that is beneficial for detoxification is yoga. By manipulating your body into different poses, it drives blood deep into your muscle tissues and holds the blood there for the duration of the pose. When you release the pose, blood that has been newly aerated by the lungs rushes in, helping to flush the old blood out. Deep breathing is also a component of yoga, which helps eliminate toxins from the blood.

Skin Brushing

In addition to eating detoxifying foods and drinking plenty of water, skin brushing can also help increase your body's natural detoxification ability. Skin brushing is quick and easy and is an incredibly effective detox tool that you can implement at home. All you need to incorporate this technique into your detox routine is a natural bristle brush.

Skin brushing is typically done with a dry brush and it is safe to do on a daily basis. To start, hold the brush in your hand and rub it gently over your skin in small circular motions. You may want to start with your feet and work your way up over your lower legs and thighs. When you reach your upper body, raise one arm at a time in the air and brush down toward your armpit. To brush your stomach and chest, brush toward your heart. Do not forget to brush your armpits as well—this is where many of your lymphatic nodes are concentrated. Avoid brushing the skin on your face, but feel free to include your neck and shoulders.

The Beauty | **Detox Diet**

Skin brushing can help increase your body's natural detoxification ability. It is quick and easy and is an incredibly effective detox tool you can implement at home.

When you first start your skin-brushing regimen, your skin may be sensitive in certain areas. Avoid brushing over cuts and bruises to prevent your skin from becoming irritated. Over time, your skin will become more resilient and it will be able to withstand more vigorous scrubbing. The entire process should take about five minutes, after which you should take a hot shower to rinse away the dead cells. In a matter of days or weeks, you should begin to notice improvements; your skin may appear more supple and radiant. Skin brushing may also reduce the appearance of cellulite.

Benefits of skin brushing may include:

- Enhancing lymphatic flow
- Exfoliating pores
- Improving cellular regeneration
- Increasing the resilience of skin
- Reducing the appearance of cellulite
- Removing dead skin cells
- Stimulating circulation and blood flow

Deep-Breathing Exercises

As you already know, your lungs are instrumental in eliminating toxins from your body. The more deeply you breathe, the more carbon dioxide you will exhale, and thus, the more toxins you will expel. Gas exchanges in the body play a significant role in detoxification. As you take oxygen into your lungs, it passes into the blood and moves throughout the body. As blood travels through your body, cells absorb the oxygen in exchange for metabolic waste (carbon dioxide). The blood eventually makes its way back to the lungs where it exchanges carbon dioxide for oxygen.

Spending just a few minutes a day
performing one or more of the following
exercises can boost your detox and help
you relieve stress and anxiety. By relaxing
for a few minutes, taking your focus
off the stressors of your daily life,
you can detox not only your body
but your mind as well.

Deep-breathing exercises improve the oxygenation of your blood. Many people tend to breathe at a fairly shallow level, especially when exercising. By concentrating on these simple exercises, you can stimulate larger portions of your lungs and increase their detoxification power. Try the following breathing exercises.

Exercise 1

1. Sit on the floor in a position you find comfortable—fold your legs in front of you or bend your knees, placing your feet flat on the floor.

2. Close your eyes and try to relax your body, keeping your spine straight.

3. Let your shoulders relax and fall.

4. Release any tension in your face and jaw.

5. Focus on taking even, regular breaths—feel the rise and fall of your chest and abdomen.

6. Continue the exercise for several minutes.

Exercise 2

1. Sit on the floor in a position you find comfortable—fold your legs in front of you or bend your knees, placing your feet flat on the floor.

2. Close your eyes and try to relax your body, keeping your spine straight.

3. Breathe in over a count of seven, then hold your breath for seven counts.

4. Exhale slowly for a count of seven. (If you cannot make it to seven seconds at first, you can use a lower number.)

5. Try breathing in through your nose and out through your mouth—if that is uncomfortable, try the reverse.

6. Focus your attention on your breathing. Do not become distracted by thoughts.

7. Continue the exercise for several minutes.

Exercise 3

1. Lie down flat on your back with your arms at your sides.

2. Breathe in slowly, allowing your abdomen to expand.

3. Exhale slowly through your nose, pulling your abdominal muscles in as you exhale. This will help push the air out of the deepest parts of your lungs.

4. Continue the exercise for several minutes.

Exercise 4

1. Lie down flat on your back with your arms at your sides.

2. Exhale as much air as you can without straining. Count the number of seconds over which you exhale.

3. Squeeze the muscles in your chest and abdomen as you exhale.

4. When you can exhale no further, inhale and repeat the process.

5. Continue the exercise for several minutes.

Exercise 5

1. Sit or lie down in a position you find comfortable and close your eyes.

2. Imagine that your lungs are divided into two sections—one upper and one lower.

3. Inhale deeply, filling the lower section of your lungs (your abdomen) with air.

4. Continue to inhale, filling the upper section (your chest).

5. Reverse the process for exhaling. Start by deflating your chest and end with the abdomen.

These breathing exercises can be incorporated into your life very easily. Spending just a few minutes a day performing one or more of these can boost your detox and help you relieve stress and anxiety. By relaxing for a few minutes, taking your focus off the stressors of your daily life, you can detox not only your body but your mind as well.

Massage for Detox

Your lymphatic system is part of your circulatory system, and it serves to carry lymph fluid toward your heart. As part of its daily function, your lymphatic system serves as a pathway for plasma that has been filtered out of the blood through capillary filtration to be returned to the blood. This is an important part of detoxification, and one way to enhance it is through massage. A form of massage called manual lymphatic drainage (MLD) is designed to stimulate your lymphatic system using gentle strokes that encourage the lymphatic system to eliminate waste products, including toxins and bacteria.

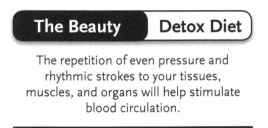

The Beauty **Detox Diet**

The repetition of even pressure and rhythmic strokes to your tissues, muscles, and organs will help stimulate blood circulation.

The MLD massage technique was developed by physical therapists in the early 1930s, and it continues to be popular today. In addition to enhancing the detoxification benefits of massage, MLD may also help promote the healing of scar tissue, clear areas of swelling or puffiness, and speed up post-operative healing. It is possible to administer your own MLD massage at home. To do so, position your fingers on either side of your neck below your ears. Gently massage your skin down toward the back of your neck. Repeat the motion ten times, repositioning your fingers slightly lower below your ear each time. Next, position your fingers on either side of your neck at the top of the shoulders. Massage your skin toward the collarbone and repeat this motion five times.

Other types of massage such as Swedish massage and deep tissue massage can also be beneficial for detox. The repetition of even pressure and rhythmic strokes to your tissues, muscles, and organs will help stimulate blood circulation. One way to think of it is that when pressure is applied, the toxins are squeezed out and released into your circulatory system so they can be eliminated. In addition to boosting your detox benefits, massage can also help with soreness, stiffness, and recovery from injury.

The Beauty   Detox Diet

Take a hot bath once in a while to help yourself relax and to boost the cleansing effects of your detox. Add a cup of Epsom salts to the bath to increase your body's absorption of magnesium. This essential mineral helps to neutralize acidic toxins in the body and also helps relax your muscles.

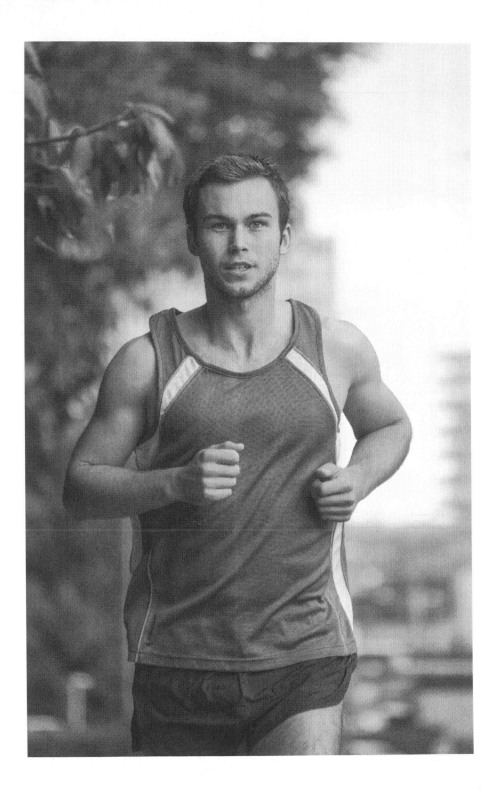

6

10 TIPS FOR BEAUTY DETOX SUCCESS

As you now know, there are a variety of factors that play into a successful beauty detox. Not only do you need to eliminate processed foods from your diet and limit your exposure to environmental toxins, but you may also need to make some changes to your everyday life. In this chapter, you will find ten beauty detox tips that sum up some of the most pertinent information you've already learned and that will help you transition into and stick with your beauty detox diet.

1. Take a moment to truly think about the way you look and feel. Many people, though they are able to perform daily activities with few problems, feel as if they aren't quite living up to their potential. If you feel like you could stand to have more energy or vitality, the beauty detox diet may be what you need. What makes the beauty detox diet unique is that it is a holistic program that doesn't just target weight loss; it also promotes healthy digestion, elimination of toxins, and improved hair and skin health.

2. After learning the dangers of daily toxins, you may find it beneficial to perform a review of your own diet and use of commercial products. Review the following list and check off the items you use on a regular basis. You may be surprised by how many potential sources of toxins you incorporate into your daily life.

☐ Alcohol

☐ Artificial sweeteners

☐ Bleached flour

☐ Caffeinated beverages

☐ Candy/sweets

☐ Canned foods

☐ Cologne/perfume

☐ Commercially raised meat

☐ Fast food

☐ Fish

☐ Frozen meals

☐ Hair products

☐ Herbicides/weed killer

☐ Household cleaners

☐ Indoor insecticides

☐ Insect repellant

☐ Laundry detergent

☐ Lotions/skin products

☐ Makeup

☐ Non-organic (conventional) produce

☐ Over-the-counter drugs

☐ Packaged meats

☐ Plastic containers

☐ Prescription medications

☐ Red meat

☐ Refined sugar

☐ Soda, juice drinks, etc.

3. Having made it this far into the book, you may be feeling guilty about all of the bad habits you have accumulated over the years. Before you go any further with the beauty detox diet, you may find it helpful to take a moment to think about all the *good* health and beauty habits you have. Habits such as getting enough sleep, engaging in regular exercise, eating plenty of vegetables, and limiting your intake of high-fat foods will help you achieve success in the beauty detox diet.

4. Remember, the recipes in this book are designed to help you transition into a cleaner, reduced-calorie diet. You will not find typical breakfast/lunch/dinner meal plans in this book. Instead, there are a variety of recipes that you can integrate into your meal repertoire to boost your beauty detox. Don't be afraid to make alterations to the recipes so they better suit your tastes.

5. The beauty detox diet is not a quick fix; it is a *process* designed to improve your overall health and wellness by cleansing your body of accumulated toxins. It took time for toxins to build up in your organs, muscles, and tissues, so you cannot expect to eliminate them immediately. Do not be discouraged if you aren't seeing results as quickly as you would like or if you briefly lapse into old habits. Change is difficult, and you should not beat yourself up over mistakes. Simply realize that tomorrow is a new day and a new chance to stick to the beauty detox diet.

6. Don't be afraid to try out some of the additional detox tricks mentioned in this book. Many people are squeamish about the idea of going on a natural colon detox or having an enema, but these procedures can greatly boost the effects of your detox diet. The goal of the beauty detox diet is to cleanse your system, and these are simply another way to do that. If you still aren't sure whether an enema might be a good choice for you, speak

to your primary care physician about the procedure. Note that in some states, businesses that provide these services operate illegally. Research the laws in your area, and find a reputable professional if you choose to proceed.

7. In modern Western cultures, many people spend their lives rushing from place to place, completing tasks as quickly as humanly possible. This rushed lifestyle may lead to a great deal of productivity, but it can also be extremely stressful. You may not realize it, but stress has an impact on your entire body. It can affect your sleep habits, your mood, and even the efficiency with which your body processes and absorbs nutrients. Learning to slow down and take a breath once in a while is an important part of the beauty detox diet.

8. After a long, stressful day at work, you may often find yourself just wanting to relax and unwind once you get home. Unfortunately, your home may be a toxic environment that adds to your daily toxin load. To achieve the greatest benefit through your beauty detox diet, you should also detoxify your home and work environments. Start by opening the windows to let in some fresh air, and swap out commercial chemicals and cleaning products for "green" options. Keep your house clean by mopping and vacuuming at least once a week, and ensure proper ventilation in damp areas to prevent mold. Make an effort to reduce your use of plastic, and consider installing a water filter.

9. One element of the beauty detox diet that people are apt to forget is exercise. While you do not need to run six miles every day or spend an hour in the gym every morning, incorporating some moderate exercise into your routine will greatly improve your detox benefits. Even simple motions like walking or stretching

can increase blood circulation throughout your body and speed up your breathing. Both of these effects serve to flush toxins from the body more quickly. Proper blood flow to your organs and tissues will ensure that they efficiently filter toxins out of your blood and eliminate them from your body.

10. Finally, don't let other people drag you down. In a culture bursting with fad diets and slim-quick schemes, some people may not understand that the beauty detox diet is unique. If you are serious about cleansing your body and improving your overall health and beauty, make an effort to keep a positive attitude. Surround yourself with supportive friends and family so they can offer you the encouragement you need and share the joys of the success you deserve.

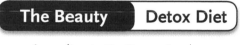

The Beauty   **Detox Diet**

According to Dr. Steven Arculeo
(2009), "losing weight will be difficult,
if not impossible, without removing
[accumulated toxins]."

PART 2
Beautiful Recipes

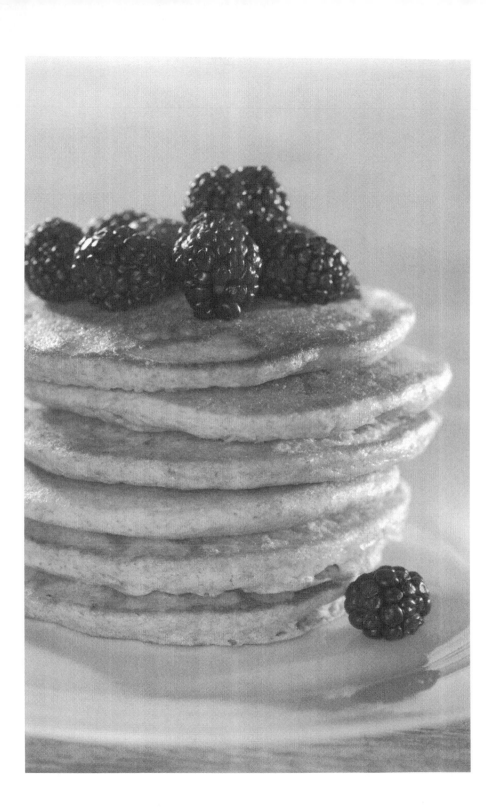

7

BEAUTIFUL WAYS TO START YOUR DAY

You may have heard it said by various health professionals that breakfast is the most important meal of the day. Skipping breakfast can not only limit your weight loss, it could also interfere with your detox. For your body to flush out toxins, it needs food for fuel and water for hydration. The recipes in this section are sure to satisfy your morning hunger and jump-start your day of detoxing.

Pumpkin Almond-Flour Pancakes

Calories: 90 per pancake

Almond flour is an excellent substitute for wheat-based flour, and this recipe is all the proof you need. The combination of pureed pumpkin and pumpkin pie spice will have you wondering whether these pancakes are more of a dessert than a breakfast.

- 1⅓ cups blanched almond flour
- ½ teaspoon baking soda
- Pinch of salt
- ½ cup pumpkin puree
- 3 large eggs, separated
- 2 tablespoons coconut oil
- 1 tablespoon raw honey
- 1 teaspoon almond extract
- 1 teaspoon pumpkin pie spice
- Cooking oil for greasing
- Maple syrup (optional)

1. Whisk together the almond flour, baking soda, and salt in a small bowl.

2. In a mixing bowl, beat together the pumpkin puree, egg yolks, and coconut oil.

3. Beat in the honey, almond extract, and pumpkin pie spice.

4. Add the dry ingredients to the pumpkin mixture and whisk until smooth.

5. In a separate bowl, beat the egg whites until they are frothy.

6. Fold the egg whites into the pancake batter, stirring until just combined.

7. Grease a large nonstick skillet with cooking oil and heat it over medium heat.

8. Spoon the batter onto the skillet using a ¼-cup measure.

9. Cook the pancakes until the batter begins to bubble on the surface, about 2 minutes.

10. Carefully flip the pancakes using a spatula and cook them for 1–2 minutes until the underside is browned.

11. Transfer the pancakes to a plate and repeat the process with the remaining batter.

12. Serve the pancakes hot and drizzle with maple syrup, if desired.

Makes about 12 pancakes.

Coconut Walnut Granola

Calories: 360 per ½-cup serving

If a piece of fruit or a muffin simply won't satisfy you, this coconut walnut granola is a hearty, filling breakfast option. Full of fiber and protein, this will keep you energized all morning.

- 2 cups rolled oats
- ½ cup chopped walnuts
- ¼ cup unsweetened flaked coconut
- 1 tablespoon ground flaxseed

- ⅓ cup raw honey
- 3 tablespoons coconut oil
- ½ teaspoon coconut extract
- ¼ teaspoon salt

---

1. Preheat oven to 300 degrees F and line a rimmed baking sheet with parchment paper.

2. Combine the rolled oats, walnuts, coconut, and flaxseed in a large mixing bowl.

3. Whisk together the remaining ingredients and pour it over the ingredients in the bowl.

4. Mix the granola by hand until everything is evenly coated.

5. Spread the granola evenly on the prepared baking sheet and bake for 10 minutes.

6. Stir the granola and then bake for another 10 minutes or until it is lightly browned.

7. Allow the granola to cool completely before storing in an airtight container.

Serves 4–5.

Lemon Coconut Muffins

Calories: 210 per muffin

Coconuts contain healthful fatty acids that boost your body's energy while also helping to cleanse toxins from your system.

- 1 cup rice flour
- ½ cup blanched almond flour
- ¼ cup arrowroot powder
- 1 tablespoon baking powder
- 1 teaspoon xanthan gum
- Pinch of salt
- 3 large eggs
- 3 tablespoons fresh lemon juice
- 1 tablespoon lemon zest
- ¾ cup unsweetened coconut milk
- ¼ cup agave nectar
- ¼ cup coconut oil, melted
- ½ cup unsweetened flaked coconut

1. Preheat oven to 350 degrees F and line a regular muffin pan with paper liners.

2. Whisk together the rice flour, almond flour, arrowroot powder, baking powder, xanthan gum, and salt in a mixing bowl.

3. In a separate bowl, beat together the eggs, lemon juice, lemon zest, and coconut milk.

4. Whisk the agave and coconut oil into the egg mixture until smooth.

5. Gradually whisk the dry ingredients into the wet until the batter is smooth and free of lumps.

6. Fold in the flaked coconut.

7. Spoon the batter into the prepared pan, filling each muffin cup about two-thirds full.

8. Bake the muffins for 25 minutes or until a knife inserted in the center comes out clean.

9. Cool the muffins in the pan for 5 minutes before turning out to serve.

Makes 12 muffins.

Apple Cinnamon Rolled Oats

Calories: 220 per ½-cup serving

This recipe is better than any oatmeal you've ever eaten from a packet. Made with crisp apples, organic apple juice, and ground cinnamon, this is a breakfast that will have you waking up early.

- 2 medium apples, cored and chopped
- 2 cups water
- ½ cup organic apple juice
- 1⅓ cups rolled oats
- 2 teaspoons ground cinnamon
- ¼ teaspoon ground nutmeg
- 2 cups unsweetened almond milk

1. Place the apples in a large saucepan and stir in the water and apple juice.

2. Bring the mixture to a boil, and then stir in the rolled oats, cinnamon, and nutmeg.

3. Bring the mixture to a boil again and then reduce the heat to low.

4. Simmer the oats until thickened, about 3–5 minutes.

5. Spoon the mixture into bowls and serve with almond milk.

Serves 4.

Silver Dollar Pancakes

Calories: 65 per pancake

Looking for a simple but satisfying breakfast? These silver dollar pancakes are just the thing—perfect for a quick family meal, or save the batter and enjoy it yourself all week.

- ¼ cup unsweetened coconut milk
- 2 tablespoons raw honey
- 1 tablespoon vanilla extract
- 3 large eggs
- 1½ cups almond flour
- ½ teaspoon baking soda
- Pinch of salt
- Cooking oil for greasing

---

1. Combine the coconut milk, honey, vanilla extract, and eggs in a mixing bowl. Beat until well combined.

2. Combine the dry ingredients in a separate bowl and stir well.

3. Gradually beat the dry ingredients into the wet until the batter is smooth.

4. Heat a nonstick skillet over medium heat and grease with cooking oil.

5. Use a tablespoon to scoop the batter onto the skillet in silver-dollar-sized circles. Cook the pancakes for 1 minute or until the batter begins to bubble.

6. Flip the pancakes using a spatula and cook until lightly browned on the underside.

7. Transfer the pancakes to a plate and serve hot.

Serves 4.

Blueberry Walnut Quinoa Casserole

Calories: 280 per ½-cup serving

This recipe is packed with detox ingredients, not to mention a delicious flavor. Blueberries are loaded with antioxidants, while walnuts contain omega-3 fatty acids. What more could you ask for in a breakfast?

- 1 cup dry quinoa
- 2 cups water
- Cooking oil for greasing
- 1½ cups unsweetened coconut milk
- 1 cup pitted dates
- ½ cup almond meal
- ½ cup chopped walnuts
- ½ cup unsweetened applesauce
- 1 tablespoon ground cinnamon
- Pinch of salt
- 1 cup fresh blueberries

1. Place the quinoa in a mesh sieve and rinse thoroughly with fresh water.

2. Transfer the quinoa to a small saucepan and add the water. Bring the quinoa to a boil and then reduce the heat and simmer, covered, for 15–20 minutes or until the water has been absorbed. Remove the quinoa from the heat and let sit for 5 minutes.

3. Preheat oven to 350 degrees F and lightly grease a square glass baking dish with cooking oil.

4. Combine the coconut milk, dates, almond meal, walnuts, applesauce, cinnamon, and salt in a blender until smooth.

5. Pour the blended mixture into a bowl, stir in the quinoa, and fold in the blueberries.

6. Spoon the mixture into the prepared dish and bake for about 1 hour or until the casserole is set.

7. Cool for 1 hour before serving.

Serves 8.

Sweet Potato Breakfast Hash

Calories: 240 per 1-cup serving

Sweet potatoes are loaded with health benefits, including complex carbohydrates, dietary fiber, and vitamin A. Additionally, sweet potatoes contain magnesium, which helps regulate blood sugar levels, and vitamin C, which helps reduce inflammation.

- 2 medium sweet potatoes, diced
- 1 tablespoon olive oil
- 1 teaspoon salt
- ½ teaspoon freshly ground black pepper
- ½ teaspoon paprika
- 2 green onions, sliced

1. Place the sweet potatoes in a mixing bowl.

2. Add the olive oil, salt, pepper, and paprika. Toss to coat.

3. Heat a skillet over medium heat and add the sweet potato mixture.

4. Cook, stirring for 8–10 minutes until the sweet potatoes are lightly browned.

5. Add the green onions and stir to combine.

6. Cook for 1 minute, stirring, and then spoon onto plates to serve.

Serves 2.

Tropical Fruit Salad

Calories: 150 per 1-cup serving

If you aren't much of a morning person, this tropical fruit salad may be the quick, light breakfast you are looking for. Toss it together early in the week and enjoy it every morning before you run out the door.

- 2 cups chopped pineapple
- 2 ripe kiwis, peeled and chopped
- 1 mango, peeled and chopped
- 1 banana, peeled and chopped
- 1 orange, peeled and chopped
- 1 tablespoon raw honey
- Pinch of cinnamon

1. Combine all of the chopped fruit in a large mixing bowl.

2. Drizzle the honey and sprinkle the cinnamon over the fruit and then toss until well combined.

3. Transfer the fruit to a serving dish and chill until ready to serve.

Serves 4–6.

Cherry Baked Oatmeal

Calories: 300 per ¾-cup serving

Baked oatmeal is the perfect Sunday morning breakfast. It is easy to prepare and full of flavor. Try it out on your family this weekend.

- Cooking oil for greasing
- 2½ cups steel-cut oats
- 1½ teaspoons baking powder
- 1 teaspoon ground cinnamon
- Pinch of salt
- 2 large eggs
- 1 cup unsweetened almond milk
- ⅓ cup raw honey
- 1 teaspoon almond extract
- ½ cup dried cherries

1. Preheat oven to 350 degrees F and lightly grease a square glass baking dish with cooking oil.

2. Combine the steel-cut oats, baking powder, cinnamon, and salt in a mixing bowl and set aside.

3. In a separate bowl, whisk together the eggs, almond milk, honey, and almond extract.

4. Stir the oat mixture into the egg mixture until well combined.

5. Fold in the dried cherries and pour the mixture into the prepared baking dish.

6. Bake for 35 minutes or until the oats have absorbed the liquid and the top is browned.

7. Cool for 10 minutes before cutting to serve.

Serves 6–8.

Maple Raspberry Muffins

Calories: 215 per muffin

These muffins have a unique and delicious flavor that will help you start your day off right. Simply pop these in the oven, and in less than 30 minutes, you will have a healthful, wholesome breakfast.

- 1 cup rice flour
- ½ cup blanched almond flour
- ¼ cup tapioca flour
- 3 teaspoons baking powder
- 1 teaspoon xanthan gum
- Pinch of salt
- 3 large eggs
- 1 cup unsweetened almond milk
- ¼ cup maple syrup
- ¼ cup coconut oil, melted
- 1 cup raspberries

---

1. Preheat oven to 350 degrees F and line a regular muffin pan with paper liners.

2. Whisk together the flours, baking powder, xanthan gum, and salt in a large mixing bowl.

3. In a separate bowl, beat together the eggs and almond milk.

4. Whisk the maple syrup and coconut oil into the egg mixture until smooth.

5. Gradually whisk the dry ingredients into the wet until the batter is smooth and free of lumps.

6. Fold in the raspberries.

7. Spoon the batter into the prepared pan, filling each muffin cup about two-thirds full.

8. Bake the muffins for 25 minutes or until a knife inserted in the center comes out clean.

9. Cool the muffins in the pan for 5 minutes before turning out to serve.

Makes 12 muffins.

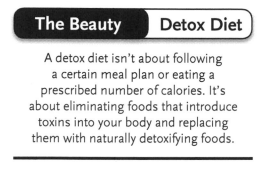

A detox diet isn't about following a certain meal plan or eating a prescribed number of calories. It's about eliminating foods that introduce toxins into your body and replacing them with naturally detoxifying foods.

Banana Coconut-Flour Pancakes

Calories: 80 per pancake

For many people, pancakes are a breakfast staple. Even though you are eliminating traditional flours from your diet, you don't have to worry about giving up a breakfast favorite. These banana pancakes are made with coconut flour, which is loaded with fiber and completely gluten-free.

- ¼ cup sifted coconut flour
- 2 teaspoons ground cinnamon
- ¼ teaspoon ground nutmeg
- 6 large eggs
- 1 cup mashed banana
- ¼ cup maple syrup, plus additional for serving (optional)
- ½ teaspoon vanilla extract
- Cooking oil for greasing

1. Whisk together the coconut flour, cinnamon, and nutmeg in a small bowl.

2. In a separate mixing bowl, beat together the eggs and banana.

3. Beat in the maple syrup and vanilla extract.

4. Add the dry ingredients to the banana mixture and whisk until smooth.

5. Grease a large nonstick skillet with cooking oil over medium heat.

6. Spoon the batter onto the skillet using a ¼ cup measure.

7. Cook the pancakes until the batter begins to bubble on the surface, about 2 minutes.

8. Carefully flip the pancakes using a spatula and cook them for 1–2 minutes until the underside is browned.

9. Transfer the pancakes to a plate and repeat the process with the remaining batter.

10. Serve the pancakes hot, drizzled with maple syrup, if desired.

Serves 4.

Baked Cinnamon Quinoa

Calories: 260 per ½-cup serving

You may have tried baked oatmeal at one point in your life, but baked quinoa may be a new concept for you. Quinoa is loaded with protein and other vital nutrients, and when baked with cinnamon and raisins, it makes a perfectly delicious breakfast.

- 1 cup dry quinoa
- 2 cups water
- Cooking oil for greasing
- 1½ cups unsweetened almond milk
- 1 cup raisins
- ½ cup unsweetened applesauce
- ½ cup flaxseeds
- ½ cup almond meal
- 1 tablespoon ground cinnamon
- Pinch of salt

1. Place the quinoa in a mesh sieve and rinse thoroughly with fresh water.

2. Transfer the quinoa to a small saucepan and add the water. Bring the quinoa to a boil and then reduce the heat and simmer, covered, for 15–20 minutes or until the water has been absorbed. Remove the quinoa from the heat and let sit for 5 minutes.

3. Preheat oven to 350 degrees F and lightly grease a square glass baking dish with cooking oil.

4. Combine the remaining ingredients in a blender until smooth.

5. Pour the blended mixture into a bowl and stir in the quinoa.

6. Spoon the mixture into the prepared dish and bake for about 1 hour or until the casserole is set.

7. Cool for 1 hour before serving.

Serves 8.

Cranberry Almond Granola

Calories: 330 per ½-cup serving

This granola is a flavorful breakfast that is sure to keep you full throughout the morning. Made with protein-packed nuts and seeds as well as antioxidant-loaded dried cranberries, this recipe is a detox powerhouse.

- 1 cup dried cranberries
- 2 cups water
- 2½ cups rolled oats
- ¾ cup raw slivered almonds
- 1 tablespoon ground flaxseed
- ⅓ cup raw honey
- ¼ tablespoon coconut oil
- ½ teaspoon almond extract
- ¼ teaspoon salt

1. Soak the cranberries in the water for 1 hour and then drain and set aside.

2. Preheat oven to 300 degrees F and line a rimmed baking sheet with parchment paper.

3. Combine the oats, almonds, flaxseed, and soaked cranberries in a large mixing bowl.

4. In another bowl, whisk together the remaining ingredients and pour over the cranberry and oat mixture.

5. Stir the mixture by hand until the granola is evenly coated.

6. Spread the granola evenly on the prepared baking sheet and bake for 10 minutes.

7. Stir the granola and then bake for another 10 minutes or until it is lightly browned.

8. Allow the granola to cool completely before serving or storing in an airtight container.

Serves 4–5.

Gluten-Free Blueberry Muffins

Calories: 200 per muffin

These blueberry muffins are as light and fluffy as any traditional muffin you have ever eaten. They have the hidden benefit, however, of being completely gluten-free.

- 1 cup rice flour
- ½ cup blanched almond flour
- ¼ cup tapioca starch
- 1 tablespoon baking powder
- 1 teaspoon xanthan gum
- Pinch of salt
- 3 large eggs
- 1 cup unsweetened almond milk
- ¼ cup raw honey
- ¼ cup coconut oil, melted
- 1 cup fresh blueberries

---

1. Preheat oven to 350 degrees F and line a regular muffin pan with paper liners.

2. Whisk together the rice flour, almond flour, tapioca starch, baking powder, xanthan gum, and salt in a mixing bowl.

3. In a separate bowl, beat together the eggs and almond milk.

4. Whisk the honey and coconut oil into the egg mixture until smooth.

5. Gradually whisk the dry ingredients into the wet until the batter is smooth and free of lumps.

6. Fold in the blueberries.

7. Spoon the batter into the prepared pan, filling each muffin cup about two thirds full.

8. Bake the muffins for 25 minutes or until a knife inserted in the center comes out clean.

9. Cool the muffins in the pan for 5 minutes before turning out to serve.

Makes 12 muffins.

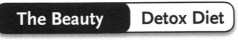

Make sure to include plenty of fiber in your detox diet because it is essential for stimulating healthy digestion. A good way to boost your fiber intake is to add some fresh berries to your morning cereal or sprinkle them on a salad at lunch.

Blackberry Almond Porridge

Calories: 280 per ¾-cup serving

A healthful blend of whole grains, nuts, and seeds, this blackberry almond porridge is a hearty nutrient-filled breakfast.

- 1 medium apple
- 1 cup unsweetened almond milk
- ½ cup rolled oats
- ¼ cup old-fashioned oats
- ¼ cup slivered almonds
- 2 tablespoons raw sunflower seeds
- 2 tablespoons ground flaxseed
- ¼ teaspoon ground cinnamon
- ½ cup fresh blackberries

1. Grate the apple into a small bowl and set aside.

2. Combine the almond milk and rolled oats in a small saucepan over low heat.

3. Stir in the old-fashioned oats, almonds, sunflower seeds, flaxseed, and cinnamon.

4. Heat the mixture, stirring, until the oats are tender.

5. Spoon the mixture into bowls and garnish with apples and blackberries.

Serves 3.

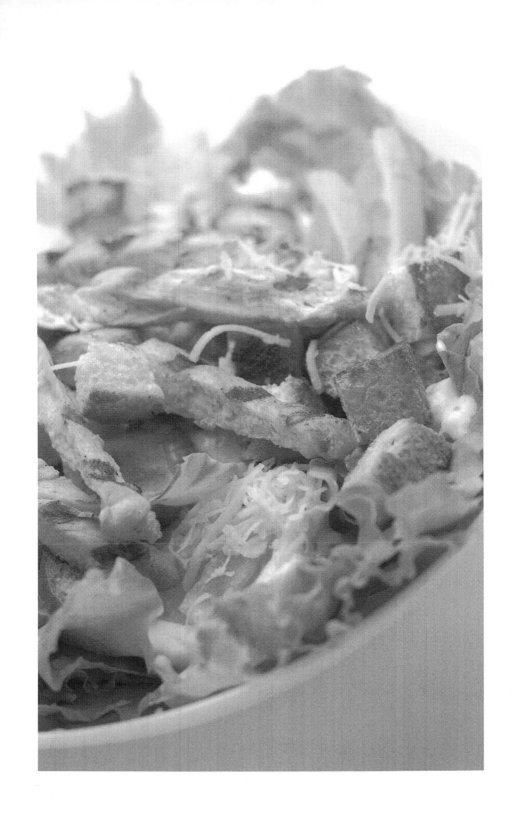

8

BEAUTIFUL ANYTIME SOUPS AND SALADS

If you have ever gone on a diet before, you may be under the impression that salads are bland, boring meals. In this section, however, you will find that salads can be full of flavor and detox power. Soups are another wonderful detox dish because they can be made with a variety of healthful fruits and vegetables, all blended into one savory dish.

Tomato Gazpacho

Calories: 200 per 1-cup serving

Lycopene, the pigment that gives tomatoes their red color, is also an antioxidant that helps cleanse the body of accumulated toxins and protects the liver from free radical damage.

- 4 ripe Roma tomatoes, halved
- 1 medium red pepper, cored and seeded
- 1 medium green pepper, cored and seeded
- 1 cucumber, seeded and quartered
- 1 small red onion, quartered
- 3 cups organic tomato juice
- ¼ cup olive oil
- ¼ cup white wine vinegar
- 1 teaspoon minced garlic
- 1 teaspoon salt
- ½ teaspoon freshly ground black pepper
- Pinch of cayenne powder (optional)

1. Place the tomatoes in a food processor and pulse several times until finely chopped. (Do not puree the tomatoes.)

2. Transfer the tomatoes to a large mixing bowl.

3. Place the red and green peppers in the food processor and pulse until finely chopped.

4. Transfer the peppers to the mixing bowl with the tomatoes.

5. Repeat this process with the cucumber and red onion, pulsing the vegetables separately and adding them to the mixing bowl.

6. Stir the tomato juice into the mixing bowl and then stir in the remaining ingredients.

7. Cover the bowl and chill for 4–6 hours.

8. Serve the soup cold, garnished with fresh herbs.

Serves 4.

Pomegranate Beet Soup

Calories: 135 per 1-cup serving

Beets are widely recognized as one of the most effective foods for detoxifying the liver. They are full of antioxidants as well as pectin, a type of fiber that helps remove toxins from the liver.

- 1 tablespoon coconut oil
- 1 teaspoon minced garlic
- 2 medium carrots, diced
- 1 medium onion, diced
- 1 small parsnip, thinly sliced

- 3 cups organic vegetable stock
- 1 cup sliced beet
- 1 pomegranate

---

1. Heat the oil in a stockpot over medium heat.

2. Stir in the garlic, carrots, onion, and parsnip. Cook for 5 minutes, stirring often.

3. Whisk in the vegetable stock and stir in the sliced beet.

4. Bring the mixture to a boil and then simmer for 20 minutes, until the beets are tender.

5. Remove the soup from the heat and puree it using an immersion blender.

6. Cut the pomegranate in half and juice it using a citrus juicer.

7. Whisk 2–4 tablespoons of the pomegranate juice into the soup. Serve hot.

Serves 4.

Avocado Spinach Salad with Almond Dressing

Calories: 350 per 1-cup serving

Spinach is a powerful detox food because it contains antioxidants that help flush toxins out of your system. Another significant benefit is that it contains chlorophyll, which helps absorb heavy metals and pesticides, making it easier for your body to eliminate those toxins.

For the dressing:
- ¼ cup raw almonds
- 3 tablespoons olive oil
- 2 sundried tomatoes in oil
- 2 tablespoons red wine vinegar
- 1 tablespoon fresh chopped cilantro
- 1 tablespoon fresh chopped mint
- Pinch of salt and pepper

For the salad:
- 8 cups fresh baby spinach
- 1 cup halved cherry tomatoes
- ½ small red onion, thinly sliced
- 1 ripe avocado, pitted and sliced

Make the dressing:
1. Combine all of the dressing ingredients in a blender. Blend the mixture until smooth and then set aside. Chill, if desired.

Make the salad:
1. Combine the spinach, tomatoes, and onion in a large mixing bowl.

2. Drizzle the dressing over the salad and toss to gently coat.

3. Divide the salad among four bowls.

4. Top each salad with a few slices of avocado and serve immediately.

Serves 4.

Creamy Cucumber Dill Soup

Calories: 180 per 1-cup serving

Cucumbers are a highly valuable detox food because they help restore your body to its natural alkaline state. After eating too many processed and high-fat foods, your body is likely to be acidic.

- 4 seedless cucumbers, peeled and quartered lengthwise
- 1 small red onion, diced
- 1 teaspoon minced garlic
- 1 bunch fresh dill
- 4 cups unsweetened almond milk
- 1 cup canned coconut milk
- ¾ cup fresh lemon juice
- 1 teaspoon salt
- ½ teaspoon freshly ground black pepper

---

1. Set two cucumbers aside, and then chop the others and place them in a large bowl.

2. Stir in the red onion and garlic.

3. Pick the ends from the dill and stir them into the cucumber mixture.

4. Whisk in the almond milk, coconut milk, lemon juice, salt, and pepper.

5. Transfer the mixture to a blender and puree.

6. Pour the soup into a large serving bowl.

7. Thinly slice the remaining cucumber and add to the bowl.

8. Cover the bowl and chill for 2 hours before serving.

Serves 8.

Cranberry Quinoa Salad

Calories: 250 per 1-cup serving

Cranberries have been used medicinally by Native Americans for hundreds of years. These berries contain a variety of antioxidants as well as hippuric acid, which helps rid the body of harmful bacteria.

For the dressing:
- ½ cup water
- ¼ cup raw cashews
- 3 tablespoons fresh lemon juice
- 2 tablespoons sesame seeds or flaxseeds
- 1 tablespoon lime zest
- 1 teaspoon minced garlic
- ½ teaspoon raw honey
- ¼ teaspoon salt
- ¼ teaspoon freshly ground black pepper

For the salad:
- 1 cup dry quinoa
- 2 cups water
- 2 cups baby spinach
- 2 green onions, sliced
- ¼ cup dried cranberries

Make the dressing:

1. Combine all of the dressing ingredients in a blender.

2. Blend the mixture until smooth.

3. Add more water, if needed to thin the dressing to the desired consistency.

Make the salad:

1. Place the quinoa in a mesh sieve and rinse thoroughly with fresh water.

2. Transfer the quinoa to a small saucepan and add the water. Bring the quinoa to a boil and then reduce the heat and simmer, covered, for 15–20 minutes or until the water has been absorbed. Remove the quinoa from the heat and let sit for 5 minutes.

3. Combine the spinach, green onions, and cranberries in a large bowl.

4. Add the cooked quinoa and toss the mixture to combine.

5. Drizzle the dressing over the salad and toss to coat. Serve immediately.

Serves 4.

Roasted Potato Leek Soup

Calories: 220 per 1-cup serving

Leeks belong to the same family as garlic and onions, so they provide many of the same benefits. For example, leeks contain vital nutrients like manganese and vitamin C, and they may also help stabilize blood-sugar levels.

- 2 pounds Yukon Gold potatoes
- 2 medium leeks
- 3 tablespoons plus 1 teaspoon olive oil, divided
- 1 teaspoon minced garlic
- 5 cups organic vegetable stock
- 1 teaspoon salt
- ½ teaspoon freshly ground black pepper
- 1 small onion, diced
- 1 cup light canned coconut milk

1. Preheat oven to 375 degrees F.

2. Wash and peel the potatoes and then cut them into 1-inch chunks.

3. Chop the dark green portions off the leeks and discard them. Dice the remaining white and light-green parts.

4. Combine the potatoes and leeks in a large mixing bowl and toss with 2 tablespoons of olive oil.

5. Arrange the potatoes and leeks on a large baking sheet and roast for 20 minutes.

6. Stir the potatoes and leeks and then roast for an additional 15–20 minutes until the potatoes are tender.

7. Heat 1 tablespoon of oil in a large stockpot over medium heat.

8. Stir in the garlic and cook for 1 minute.

9. Add the roasted potatoes and leeks and then stir in the vegetable stock, salt, and pepper.

10. Bring the mixture to a boil and then reduce the heat and simmer, covered, for 45 minutes.

11. Meanwhile, heat the remaining 1 teaspoon of oil in a skillet over medium-high heat.

12. Stir in the onions and cook until tender and then set aside.

13. Remove the soup from the heat and puree with an immersion blender.

14. Return the soup to the heat and whisk in the coconut milk.

15. Cook for 5 minutes or until heated through and then ladle into bowls and garnish with sautéed onions to serve.

Serves 6.

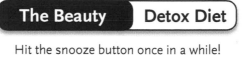

The Beauty   Detox Diet

Hit the snooze button once in a while! Getting enough sleep is extremely important for a successful detox. Make sure you give yourself at least seven hours to rest each night, and think about incorporating some other relaxation principles such as yoga or meditation into your daily routine.

Tomato Arugula Salad with Pesto Dressing

Calories: 250 per 1-cup serving

Arugula is a lettuce that is often overlooked but contains a variety of healthful benefits. In addition to its fiber content, arugula also contains glucosinolates, which help reduce your risk for cancer.

For the dressing:
- ¼ cup fresh basil leaves
- 1½ tablespoons olive oil
- 4 tablespoons pine nuts
- ½ tablespoon balsamic vinegar
- 1 clove garlic, minced

For the salad:
- 6 cups fresh arugula
- 1 cup cherry tomatoes, halved
- ¼ cup toasted pine nuts

Make the dressing:
1. Combine all of the dressing ingredients in a food processor.
2. Blend until smooth and creamy, adding more olive oil if needed to thin to the desired consistency.

Make the salad:
1. Place the arugula in a bowl and add the dressing.
2. Toss to coat the arugula and then divide it among four bowls.
3. Top each salad with cherry tomatoes and 1 tablespoon pine nuts to serve.

Serves 4.

Creamy Carrot Ginger Soup

Calories: 200 per 1-cup serving

Carrots are incredibly nutritious, which makes them an excellent addition to any detox diet. These vegetables contain a variety of minerals and antioxidants, helping to detox the liver and encourage healthy digestion.

- 3½ pounds carrots
- 2 tablespoons coconut oil
- 1 tablespoon fresh grated ginger
- 2 teaspoons minced garlic
- 1 cup chopped onion
- 6 cups organic vegetable stock
- 1 teaspoon salt
- ½ teaspoon freshly ground black pepper

1. Wash the carrots and chop them coarsely.

2. Heat the coconut oil in a large stockpot over medium heat.

3. Stir in the ginger and garlic and cook for 1 minute.

4. Add the onion and stir well. Cook for 5 minutes and then stir in the carrots. Cook for 20–25 minutes until the carrots are tender.

5. Whisk in the remaining ingredients and simmer the soup for 30 minutes.

6. Remove the soup from the heat and puree with an immersion blender.

Serves 6.

Toasted Almond Quinoa Salad

Calories: 370 per 1-cup serving

This quinoa salad is packed with nutritious ingredients. Not only do you benefit from the protein and heart-healthful fats of the toasted almonds, but you also receive a variety of detox vitamins and minerals from the quinoa, tomatoes, and cranberries.

- 1 cup dry quinoa
- 2 cups water
- 2 tablespoons coconut oil
- 1 cup halved cherry tomatoes
- ½ cup toasted almonds, chopped
- ½ cup dried cranberries
- ½ cup diced red onion
- ½ cup diced celery
- 1 carrot, diced
- ¼ cup fresh chopped mint leaves
- ¼ cup fresh chopped cilantro
- 2 tablespoons fresh lemon juice
- ½ teaspoon salt
- ¼ teaspoon freshly ground black pepper

1. Place the quinoa in a mesh sieve and rinse thoroughly with fresh water.

2. Transfer the quinoa to a small saucepan and add the water. Bring the quinoa to a boil and then reduce the heat and simmer, covered, for 15–20 minutes or until the water has been absorbed. Remove the quinoa from the heat and let sit for 2 minutes.

3. Stir in the oil and then set aside to cool.

4. Combine the remaining ingredients in a large mixing bowl.

5. Stir in the cooled quinoa and toss to combine. Serve immediately.

Serves 6.

Mango Avocado Gazpacho

Calories: 270 per 1-cup serving

This gazpacho is a unique and refreshing recipe perfect for a hot summer day. Avocado is an excellent source of heart-healthful fats, and it contains high levels of soluble and insoluble fiber, which helps to cleanse the colon.

- 2 ripe mangos, pitted and chopped
- 2 jalapeño peppers, seeded and minced
- 1 tart apple, cored and chopped
- 1 stalk celery, chopped
- ½ red pepper, seeded and chopped
- ⅔ cup orange juice
- 2 tablespoons fresh lime juice
- 1 tablespoon rice vinegar
- 1 tablespoon fresh grated ginger
- 1 teaspoon salt
- Pinch of ground cumin
- 1 seedless cucumber, peeled and diced
- 1 ripe avocado, pitted and sliced
- 3 tablespoons fresh chopped cilantro

1. Combine the first 11 ingredients in a food processor and blend until smooth and pureed. (If you don't have a large enough food processor, you may need to do this in several batches.)

2. Pour the gazpacho into a container and stir in the diced cucumber.

3. Cover the container and chill overnight.

4. Ladle the soup into bowls and top with one or two slices of fresh avocado.

5. Garnish with chopped cilantro to serve.

Serves 6.

Greek Detox Salad

Calories: 280 per 1-cup serving

The star ingredient in this detox recipe is artichoke hearts. Artichokes contain high levels of cynarin, a chemical that boosts bile production and liver function to help flush out toxins.

- 6 cups fresh arugula
- 2 celery stalks, sliced
- 1 small seedless cucumber, thinly sliced
- ½ small red onion, thinly sliced
- 1 (14-ounce) can artichoke hearts, drained and coarsely chopped
- 2 tablespoons olive oil
- 2 tablespoons fresh lemon juice
- 1 teaspoon salt
- ½ teaspoon freshly ground black pepper

1. Combine the arugula, celery, cucumber, and onion in a large bowl. Toss the ingredients to combine and then divide among four plates.

2. Sprinkle the artichoke hearts over the prepared salads.

3. Whisk together the remaining ingredients and drizzle over the salads to serve.

Serves 4.

Asparagus Quinoa Soup

Calories: 420 per 1-cup serving

Quinoa is a gluten-free grain that is loaded with health benefits. In addition to being high in protein and dietary fiber, quinoa also helps to cleanse your digestive tract.

- 1 tablespoon olive oil
- 1 teaspoon minced garlic
- 2 large onions, chopped or sliced
- 2 tablespoons plus 3 cups water, divided
- 1 bunch asparagus, chopped
- ¼ cup dry quinoa
- 1 bunch baby spinach, chopped
- 4 cups organic vegetable stock
- ¼ teaspoon ground turmeric
- 1 tablespoon fresh lemon juice

1. Heat the olive oil in a skillet over medium-high heat.

2. Stir in the garlic and onions and cook for 5 minutes or until the onions begin to brown.

3. Add 2 tablespoons of water to the pan and then cover and reduce the heat to low.

4. Simmer the onions for 25 minutes or until completely caramelized.

5. Meanwhile, bring a large pot of lightly salted water to boil.

6. Add the chopped asparagus and cook for 1 minute.

7. Drain the asparagus and rinse with cold water. Set the asparagus aside.

8. In a large saucepan, combined the rinsed quinoa with ¾ cup of water.

9. Bring the water to a boil and then reduce the heat and simmer, covered, for about 15 minutes until the quinoa is tender.

10. Stir the spinach into the saucepan and cook for 5 minutes until just wilted.

11. Add the caramelized onions and garlic, cooked asparagus, vegetable stock, and turmeric.

12. Bring the mixture to a simmer and then cover and cook for 5 minutes more.

13. Puree the soup with an immersion blender until smooth.

14. Stir in the lemon juice and serve the soup hot.

Serves 8.

Blackberry Scallion Salad

Calories: 190 per 1-cup serving

Blackberries are full of delicious flavor and they are also packed with antioxidants, dietary fiber, and vitamin C. Combined with fresh mint, lemon juice, and spring greens, this salad is loaded with detox power.

For the dressing:
- Juice of 1 lemon
- 2 tablespoons red wine vinegar
- 2 tablespoons sesame seeds
- 1 tablespoon olive oil
- ½ teaspoon freshly ground black pepper
- ¼ teaspoon salt
- ¼ teaspoon raw honey

For the salad:
- 4 cups fresh spring greens
- 2 cups fresh blackberries
- 1 small scallion, thinly sliced
- 1 tablespoon fresh chopped mint
- 1 tablespoon lemon zest

Make the dressing:

1. Whisk together all of the dressing ingredients in a small bowl and set aside.

Make the salad:

1. Combine all of the salad ingredients in a large mixing bowl.

2. Drizzle the dressing over the salad and toss to coat.

3. Serve immediately or chill before serving.

Serves 4.

Butternut Squash Soup

Calories: 140 per 1-cup serving

Butternut squash contains complex carbohydrates that break down in your body slowly, giving you long-lasting energy. Squash also contains a variety of vitamins and minerals, such as beta-carotene, which improves hair and skin health.

- 1 large butternut squash
- 1 tablespoon coconut oil
- 1 teaspoon minced garlic
- 2 teaspoons fresh chopped thyme
- 2 medium yellow onions, chopped
- 2 large celery sticks, sliced
- 4 cups organic vegetable stock
- ½ teaspoon salt
- ¼ teaspoon freshly ground black pepper
- Fresh chopped chives

1. Use a sharp knife to cut the squash in half. Scoop out the seeds with a spoon and peel off the skin. Chop the flesh into 1-inch chunks and set aside.

2. Heat the coconut oil in a large stockpot over medium heat and then stir in the garlic and thyme.

3. Cook for 1 minute and then add the onion and celery.

4. Stir in the butternut squash and cook for 5 minutes.

5. Whisk in the remaining ingredients except for the chives, and bring the mixture to a boil.

6. Simmer for 20 minutes until the squash is tender.

7. Remove from the heat and puree the soup with an immersion blender.

8. Ladle the soup into bowls and garnish with chopped chives to serve.

Serves 4.

Tomato Bean Salad

Calories: 230 per ¾-cup serving

This salad is perfect for summer picnics and potluck dinners. Made with just a few simple ingredients, it's full of nutrition and flavor—a great addition to any detox diet.

For the dressing:
- ¼ cup olive oil
- 1 teaspoon minced garlic
- 1 small sprig fresh rosemary
- ¼ cup fresh lemon juice
- 1 teaspoon lime zest
- ½ teaspoon salt
- ½ teaspoon freshly ground black pepper

For the salad:
- 1 (15-ounce) can white cannellini beans, rinsed and drained
- 2 cups halved cherry tomatoes
- 2 tablespoons fresh chopped mint
- 2 tablespoons fresh chopped parsley

Make the dressing:

1. Pour the olive oil into a small saucepan and add the garlic and rosemary.

2. Heat the saucepan over medium heat until the rosemary starts sizzling. Remove from the heat and allow to cool for 20 minutes.

3. Discard the rosemary and whisk the remaining ingredients into the dressing. Process the dressing in a food processor to achieve a smoother consistency, if desired.

Make the salad:

1. Combine all of the salad ingredients in a serving bowl.

2. Pour the dressing over the salad and toss to coat. Chill before serving, if desired.

Serves 6–8.

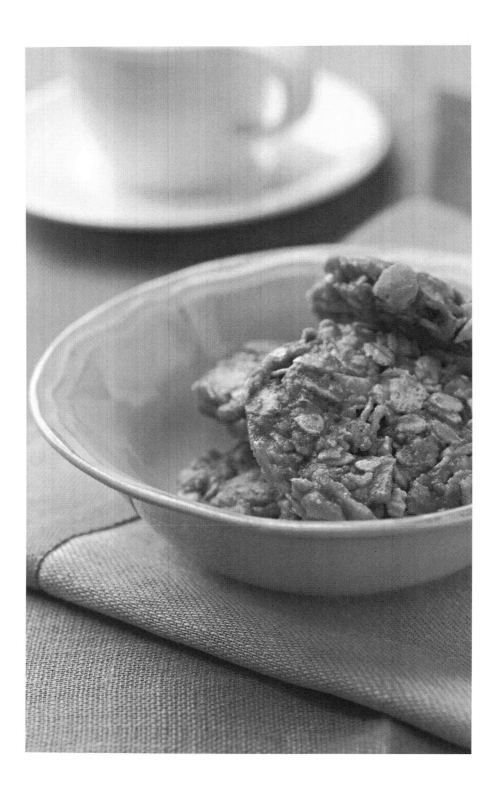

9

BEAUTIFUL DESSERTS

For many people, the word "dessert" invokes images of mile-high ice cream sundaes and monstrous slices of cake. These typical desserts are loaded with calories, processed ingredients, and toxins that will weigh you down and then some. In this section, you will find a collection of healthful (and delicious) recipes to boost your detox diet while satisfying your sweet tooth.

Strawberry Kiwi Frozen Fruit Bars

Calories: 100 per bar

Fresh fruits such as strawberry and kiwi are loaded with healthful vitamins and antioxidants. That makes this dessert both healthful and refreshing.

- 2 cups fresh sliced strawberries
- 3 fresh kiwis, peeled and sliced
- ½ cup raw honey
- 2½ tablespoons fresh lemon juice

1. Combine all of the ingredients in a food processor and blend until smooth.

2. Pour the fruit mixture into six ice pop molds.

3. Freeze the molds until the fruit bars are solid.

Makes 6 bars.

Agave Baked Bananas

Calories: 75 per banana half

If you love Bananas Foster but are looking for something a little more compatible with your detox diet, these baked bananas are perfect. Baked until tender and sweetened with agave, these bananas will hit the spot.

- 2 ripe bananas
- 1 tablespoon agave nectar
- Pinch of cinnamon

1. Preheat oven to 400 degrees F.

2. Slice the bananas in half lengthwise and remove the peels.

3. Arrange the bananas in a glass baking dish.

4. Drizzle the agave over the bananas and sprinkle with cinnamon.

5. Cover the dish with foil and bake for 10–15 minutes until tender.

Serves 4.

The Beauty Detox Diet

Avoid meals that require a long list of ingredients—even if the ingredients are healthful. The simpler your meals are, the easier they will be for your body to digest. It also means that they will have less of an impact on your blood-sugar levels, which will prevent energy fluctuations and will also help stave off weight gain.

Goji Berry Soufflés

Calories: 400 per ramekin

Goji berries are loaded with health benefits, from improving eyesight and sexual function to boosting immune system function and improving circulation. Who knew that a dessert this tasty could also be so good for you?

- 1½ cups raw cashews
- 5 cups water, divided
- 1 cup goji berries
- ¾ cup raw honey
- 3 tablespoons coconut oil, melted
- 1 teaspoon vanilla extract
- 1 teaspoon almond extract
- 1 teaspoon fresh lemon juice
- Pinch of salt

1. Place the cashews in a bowl and cover with 2 cups of water. Soak for 1–2 hours and then drain and set aside.

2. Combine the goji berries and 1 cup of water in a small bowl and soak for 15 minutes.

3. Drain the water and place the goji berries in a food processor.

4. Blend the goji berries until smooth and then strain them through a mesh sieve and discard the solids.

5. Combine the soaked cashews and blended goji berries in a blender. Add the remaining ingredients, including the remaining water, and blend until smooth and combined.

6. Pour the mixture into ramekins and freeze for 4–5 hours.

7. Submerge the frozen soufflés in a warm-water bath until loosened and then turn them out onto dessert plates to serve.

Serves 6.

Chocolate Cupcakes

Calories: 150 per cupcake

You may be surprised to find cupcakes on the list of detox desserts. The key is to use healthful ingredients like coconut flour, raw honey, and coconut oil. Combined with cocoa powder, these ingredients create the perfect chocolate cupcake.

- ¼ cup sifted coconut flour
- ¼ cup unsweetened cocoa
- ½ teaspoon baking soda
- Pinch of salt

- 4 large eggs
- 5 tablespoons raw honey
- ¼ cup coconut oil, melted

---

1. Preheat oven to 350 degrees F.

2. Line a regular muffin pan with 8 paper liners and set aside.

3. Combine the flour, cocoa, baking soda, and salt in a food processor and pulse to blend.

4. Add the remaining ingredients and pulse until the mixture is smooth and combined.

5. Spoon the batter into the prepared cups about ¼ cup at a time.

6. Bake for 15–18 minutes until a knife inserted in the center comes out clean.

7. Cool the cupcakes before serving.

Makes 8 cupcakes.

Cinnamon Poached Apples

Calories: 80 per apple

Poaching is a cooking method that many people are not familiar with. In this recipe, however, you will learn that it's a quick way to infuse fruits with delicious flavor.

- 6 cups apple juice
- 1 cinnamon stick

- 4 ripe apples, peeled and cored

---

1. Combine the apple juice and cinnamon stick in a saucepan and bring to a boil.

2. Cut the apples in half and add them to the saucepan.

3. Cover the saucepan and simmer for 7–8 minutes or until the apples are tender.

4. Remove the apples using a slotted spoon and serve hot.

Serves 4.

Balsamic Berry Mint Medley

Calories: 130 per 1-cup serving

If you are looking for a light dessert that packs plenty of flavor, this medley is just the thing. The sweetness of fresh berries blends perfectly with the balsamic vinegar, giving this recipe a unique flavor.

- 2 cups fresh sliced strawberries
- 2 cups fresh blueberries
- 1 cup fresh raspberries
- 1 cup fresh blackberries
- 2 tablespoons balsamic vinegar
- 1 tablespoon raw honey
- ¼ cup fresh mint leaves

1. Combine the berries in a mixing bowl.

2. In a separate bowl, whisk together the balsamic vinegar and honey, then drizzle it over the berries and toss to coat.

3. Let the berries sit for 45 minutes to an hour. Then toss the berries with fresh mint leaves and spoon into cups to serve.

Serves 6.

Baked Apple Crumble

Calories: 150 per ramekin

This crumble has all the flavor of a fresh apple pie without all the guilt.
Made with almond flour instead of bleached flour, and honey instead of
refined sugar, this dessert might surprise you.

- Cooking oil for greasing
- 2 cups almond flour
- 1 teaspoon ground cinnamon
- Pinch of salt
- ⅓ cup coconut oil, melted
- ¼ cup raw honey
- 2 teaspoons vanilla extract
- 5 medium apples, peeled and chopped

1. Preheat oven to 350 degrees F and lightly grease 6 small ramekins with cooking oil.

2. Combine the almond flour, cinnamon, and salt in a bowl.

3. In a separate bowl, whisk together the coconut oil, honey, and vanilla extract.

4. Gradually whisk the dry ingredients into the wet to form a smooth batter.

5. Spoon the apples into the ramekins and top with the batter.

6. Bake for 30 minutes or until the apples are tender and the topping is browned.

7. Cool for 10 minutes before serving.

Serves 6.

Hazelnut Cocoa Fudge

Calories: 130 per square

If you're in the mood for a rich, chocolaty treat, then this hazelnut cocoa fudge is just what you've been looking for. Made with raw, wholesome ingredients, you don't have to worry about this treat interfering with your detox.

- 1 cup hazelnut butter
- 1 cup unsweetened cocoa
- 1 cup raw honey
- ½ cup coconut butter
- ½ cup cocoa butter
- 1 teaspoon vanilla extract
- 1 teaspoon almond extract
- Pinch of salt

1. Combine all of the ingredients in a food processor and then blend the mixture until smooth and well combined.

2. Spoon the mixture into a parchment- or foil-lined glass dish.

3. Chill until firm and then cut into 24 squares to serve.

Serves 24.

Agave Ginger Cookies

Calories: 55 per cookie

Agave nectar is a low-glycemic natural sweetener that can be used in many of the same ways as honey. Try it in this delicious recipe for ginger cookies.

- 2½ cups almond flour
- ½ teaspoon baking soda
- ½ teaspoon ground ginger
- Pinch of salt
- 3 large eggs
- ¾ cup agave nectar
- 3 tablespoons coconut oil, melted
- 3 tablespoons fresh grated ginger
- ½ teaspoon ground cinnamon

1. Preheat oven to 350 degrees F and line a cookie sheet with parchment paper.

2. Combine the almond flour, baking soda, ground ginger, and salt in a medium bowl.

3. In a separate bowl, beat together the eggs and agave nectar.

4. Beat in the coconut oil, grated ginger, and ground cinnamon.

5. Gradually beat the dry ingredients into the wet until the dough is smooth.

6. Roll the dough into ½-inch balls by hand and arrange them on the prepared cookie sheet.

7. Bake for 10–12 minutes or until the cookies are lightly browned.

8. Cool in the pan for 3 minutes and then transfer to a wire rack to cool completely.

Makes about 5 dozen.

Vanilla Crème Parfait

Calories: 270 per ½-cup serving

For some people, giving up ice cream on a detox diet can be quite a challenge. This recipe for vanilla crème parfaits is the perfect alternative. It's full of fresh vanilla flavor and topped with your favorite fruit or nuts. What more could you ask for?

- 2 cups young coconut meat
- ¼ cup raw honey
- 2 tablespoons coconut oil
- 2 tablespoons fresh lemon juice
- ½ vanilla bean
- Pinch of salt

1. Combine the coconut meat, honey, coconut oil, and lemon juice in a food processor. Blend the ingredients until just combined.

2. Using a sharp knife, carefully cut the vanilla bean in half and split half of the bean lengthwise down the center.

3. Scrape the small black seeds from the vanilla bean into the food processor with the rest of the ingredients and then add the salt.

4. Blend until smooth and combined and then spoon into a bowl.

5. Chill for 4–6 hours or until firm. Spoon into dessert cups and top with fruit or nuts.

Serves 4.

Cinnamon Grilled Peaches

Calories: 150 per peach

If you've never eaten grilled peaches, you don't know what you are missing. These peaches are warm and tender, infused with the sweetness of honey and the flavor of cinnamon.

- Cooking oil for greasing
- 4 large ripe peaches
- 2 tablespoons raw honey
- 1 tablespoon coconut oil
- 2 teaspoons ground cinnamon

1. Preheat a grill over medium-high heat and lightly grease with cooking oil.

2. Cut the peaches in half and remove the pits.

3. Combine the honey, coconut oil, and cinnamon in a microwave-safe bowl.

4. Microwave the mixture on high for 10–15 seconds or until melted.

5. Place the peaches cut-side down on the grill and brush with the honey mixture.

6. Cook the peaches for 3–4 minutes on each side, brushing with the honey mixture several times.

7. Serve the peaches hot with extra honey glaze, if desired.

Serves 4.

Blueberry Lime Sorbet

Calories: 80 per ½-cup serving

This sorbet is the perfect treat to cool you down on a hot summer day. Best of all, it will help boost your detox as well.

- ½ cup raw honey
- 2 tablespoons fresh lime juice
- 5 cups fresh blueberries
- 1 teaspoon lime zest

---

1. Combine the honey and lime juice in a saucepan over medium heat until the honey is dissolved. Set the mixture aside to cool.

2. Place the berries in a food processor and puree.

3. Add the honey mixture and lime zest and then blend until smooth.

4. Strain the mixture through a mesh sieve and pour the strained liquid into a shallow container.

5. Freeze the sorbet until solid. When ready to serve, break the sorbet into chunks and blend in a food processor until smooth.

Serves 10–12.

Maple Oatmeal Cookies

Calories: 90 per cookie

Just because you are engaging in a detox diet doesn't mean you have to give up delicious food. These maple oatmeal cookies, for example, are less than one hundred calories each.

- 1½ cups old-fashioned oats
- 1½ cups almond flour
- 1¼ teaspoons baking powder
- 1 teaspoon ground cinnamon
- ½ teaspoon baking soda
- ½ teaspoon salt
- ¾ cup pure maple syrup
- ¼ cup coconut oil, melted
- 2 large eggs

1. Preheat oven to 350 degrees F and line a cookie sheet with parchment paper.

2. Whisk together the oats, flour, baking powder, cinnamon, baking soda, and salt in a medium bowl.

3. In a separate bowl, beat together the maple syrup, coconut oil, and eggs.

4. Gradually beat the dry ingredients into the wet until just combined.

5. Drop the dough in heaping teaspoons onto the prepared cookie sheet.

6. Bake for 8–9 minutes until the cookies are lightly browned on the edges.

7. Cool for 3 minutes in the pan and then transfer to a wire rack to cool completely.

Makes about 4 dozen.

Multilayer Frozen Fruit Cups

Calories: 100 per cup

Fresh fruit is a key component of any successful detox diet, and these frozen fruit cups are the perfect way to get your daily recommended amount.

- 2 cups water
- ½ cup raw honey
- 3 teaspoons fresh lemon juice

- 1 cup fresh strawberries
- 1 cup fresh blueberries
- 1 cup fresh raspberries
- 6 wooden ice pop sticks

---

1. Combine the water and honey in a small saucepan and cook until the honey dissolves. Stir in the lemon juice and then set aside to cool.

2. Puree the fruit in a food processor in separate batches, pouring each berry mixture into a separate bowl.

3. Divide the sweetened water evenly between the three bowls of berries, stirring to combine.

4. Spoon several tablespoons of the strawberry mixture into 6 paper cups and freeze until solid.

5. Add a few tablespoons of the blueberry mixture and stick a wooden ice pop stick in the center of each cup and freeze until solid.

6. Top the cups off with the raspberry mixture and freeze solid.

7. To serve, peel the paper away from the frozen fruit mixture.

Serves 6.

Raw Almond Gelato

Calories: 210 per ½-cup serving

This gelato is cool, refreshing, and full of detox benefits. If you are looking for a creamy treat, this recipe is sure to hit the spot.

- 1¼ cups unsweetened almond milk
- ¾ cup raw cashews
- ½ cup young coconut meat
- ½ cup raw honey
- ½ cup melted coconut butter
- 1 tablespoon almond extract
- 1 tablespoon vanilla extract
- Pinch of salt

1. Combine all of the ingredients in a food processor or blender and blend until smooth and well combined.

2. Pour the ingredients into an ice-cream maker and freeze according to the manufacturer's instructions.

Serves 2.

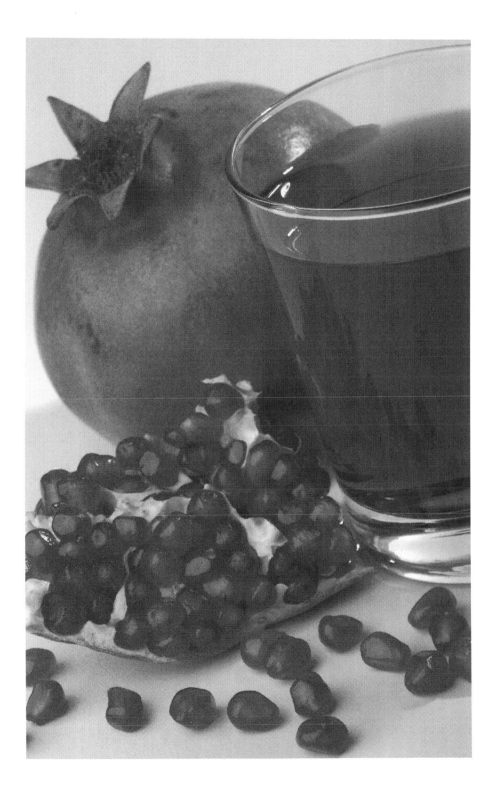

10

BEAUTIFUL JUICES AND SMOOTHIES

Juices and smoothies are perfect super foods for detoxing and cleansing your system. By using a juicer or blender, the vital nutrients in fruits and vegetables are more quickly absorbed by your body. You'll feel full and satisfied by drinking just one of these meals in a glass.

Grape Apple Kale Juice

Calories: 120 per serving (½ of recipe)

This juice recipe combines the antioxidant power of grapes and apples with nutrient-loaded kale, all in a delicious beverage. The beauty of this recipe is that you don't need a juicer to make it—all you need is a blender.

- 2 cups chopped kale leaves
- 1 cup red seedless grapes
- 1 medium apple, cored and chopped
- ½ cup water
- 2 tablespoons ground flaxseed

1. Rinse the kale well and place it in the blender.

2. Add the remaining ingredients in the order listed.

3. Pulse the mixture 2–3 times to chop the ingredients and then blend them on high speed until smooth, about 1 minute.

4. Pour the juice into 2 glasses and serve immediately.

Serves 2.

Zesty Lemon Blueberry Smoothie

Calories: 160 per serving (½ of recipe)

Lemon is an excellent food for detoxing because it contains high levels of vitamin C, which transforms harmful toxins into material that can be digested by the body. Citrus fruits like lemon also support healthful liver function.

- 2 cups frozen blueberries
- 1 cup orange juice
- 1 medium apple, cored and chopped
- 2 tablespoons fresh lemon juice
- 1 tablespoon lemon zest

1. Combine the blueberries and orange juice in a blender and blend until smooth.

2. Add the remaining ingredients and blend until smooth.

3. Pour the smoothie into 2 glasses and serve immediately.

Serves 2.

Mint Cocoa Shake

Calories: 280 per serving (½ of recipe)

Fresh herbs like mint are a valuable part of any detox diet. In this recipe, the fresh taste of mint blends perfectly with the flavors of coconut and cocoa in a cool, creamy shake.

- 2 cups unsweetened coconut milk
- ½ cup young coconut meat
- ¼ cup unsweetened cocoa

- ¼ cup raw honey
- ¼ cup fresh mint leaves
- ½ teaspoon vanilla extract

---

1. Combine all of the ingredients in a blender. Blend the mixture until smooth and then pour into 2 glasses to serve.

Serves 2.

Pomegranate Spirulina Juice

Calories: 120 per serving (½ of recipe)

Spirulina powder is made from dried algae, which is rich in protein and essential amino acids. Combining this powder with the strong flavor of pomegranates will help to neutralize the spirulina's bitter taste.

- 2 ripe pomegranates
- 1 large grapefruit, peeled and halved
- 1 large orange, peeled and halved
- 1 bunch spinach leaves
- 1 tablespoon dried spirulina powder

1. Cut the pomegranates in half and juice them using a citrus juicer. Set the juice aside.

2. Feed the grapefruit, orange, and spinach leaves through a juicer according to the manufacturer's directions.

3. Stir the spirulina powder into the juice.

4. Pour the juice into 2 glasses and pour some of the pomegranate juice into the top of each glass. Enjoy immediately.

Serves 2.

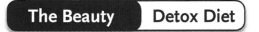

The Beauty | Detox Diet

Amp up the detox power of your meals by making each one about 70 percent vegetables. This is easier than you may think: add a side salad, a side of steamed veggies, or even a glass of fresh vegetable juice. Don't be afraid to experiment with different combinations.

Spinach Kale Strawberry Smoothie

Calories: 110 per serving (½ of recipe)

Strawberries are an excellent source of dietary fiber and healthful vitamins. These delicious berries also contain a chemical compound called phenols, which help boost the body's levels of uric acid, which is essential for detoxing.

- 1½ cups baby spinach leaves
- 1 cup chopped kale leaves
- 1 cup orange juice
- 1 cup frozen strawberries

- 2 tablespoons ground flaxseed
- 1 tablespoon raw honey (optional)

---

1. Rinse the greens well and place them in a blender. Add the orange juice and blend the mixture until smooth.

2. Add the remaining ingredients and blend until smooth.

3. Pour the smoothie into 2 glasses and serve immediately.

Serves 2.

Blueberry Mango Juice

Calories: 215 per serving (½ of recipe)

Mango contains a number of healthful vitamins and minerals as well as antioxidants. It is also a natural diuretic, which helps flush excess water and toxins from your system.

- 3 cups frozen mango chunks
- 2 cups frozen blueberries
- 2 cups unsweetened coconut milk
- 1 teaspoon almond extract
- Pinch of salt

1. Combine all of the ingredients in a blender. Blend the mixture until smooth and pour into 2 glasses to serve.

Serves 2.

Ginger Beet Juice

Calories: 120 per serving (½ of recipe)

Ginger is a flavorful spice that also helps restore healthy digestion. By stimulating the digestive system, ginger helps the body to recover from damage caused by toxins.

- 2 large carrots, chopped
- 1 medium beet, chopped
- 1 medium pear, cored and chopped
- ½ cup water
- 2 tablespoons fresh grated ginger
- Juice from 1 orange

---

1. Wash the carrots and beets and place them in a blender. Add the chopped pear, water, and ginger.

2. Juice the orange and pour into the blender.

3. Pulse the mixture 2–3 times to chop the ingredients and then blend them on high speed until smooth, about 1 minute.

4. Pour the juice into 2 glasses and serve immediately.

Serves 2.

Pineapple Banana Smoothie

Calories: 180 per serving (½ of recipe)

Pineapple is an excellent ingredient for restoring digestive health because it contains the enzyme bromelain. Pineapple also contains a number of vitamins, including vitamin C.

- 2 cups fresh chopped pineapple
- 1 large frozen banana, sliced
- 1 large carrot, chopped
- 1 cup pineapple juice
- 5–6 ice cubes
- 1 tablespoon chia seeds

1. Combine the pineapple, banana, and carrot in a blender and pulse to chop. Add the pineapple juice and blend the mixture until smooth.

2. Add the remaining ingredients and blend until smooth.

3. Pour the smoothie into 2 glasses and serve immediately.

Serves 2.

Blackberry Lemonade

Calories: 280 per serving (½ of recipe)

Blackberries are full of healthful antioxidants as well as numerous vitamins and minerals. As part of your detox diet, blackberries can also help reduce your risk for cancer.

- 3 cups water
- 1 cup fresh lemon juice
- ½ cup agave nectar
- ½ cup frozen blackberries

---

1. Whisk together the water, lemon juice, and agave nectar in a pitcher.

2. Chill the mixture until cold.

3. Slightly thaw and mash the blackberries.

4. Spoon about 2 tablespoons of the blackberries into each glass and fill with lemonade.

5. Serve immediately.

Serves 2.

Almond Sweet Potato Juice

Calories: 160 per serving (½ of recipe)

Almonds are an essential part of any detox because they contain high levels of protein and fiber, along with a number of other vital nutrients. Almonds also contain enzymes that help stimulate healthy digestion.

- 1 large sweet potato, chopped
- 1 large carrot, chopped
- 1 medium orange, peeled and sectioned
- 1 medium apple, cored and chopped
- ½ cup water
- 3 tablespoons raw almonds
- ¼ teaspoon ground ginger

1. Place the chopped sweet potato and carrot in a blender. Add the orange, apple, water, almonds, and ginger.

2. Pulse the mixture 2–3 times to chop the ingredients and then blend them on high speed until smooth, about 1 minute.

3. Pour the juice into 2 glasses and serve immediately.

Serves 2.

Black Cherry Vanilla Smoothie

Calories: 180 per serving (½ of recipe)

Cherries are an excellent source of antioxidants, which help to reduce inflammation. These can also help reduce uric acid in the joints, which, in turn, reduces oxidative stress.

- 2 cups pitted black cherries
- 1 frozen banana, sliced
- ½ cup unsweetened almond milk
- 3–4 ice cubes
- 1 tablespoon raw honey
- 1 teaspoon vanilla extract

1. Combine the cherries and banana in a blender and pulse to chop.

2. Add the almond milk and blend the mixture until smooth. Add the remaining ingredients and blend until smooth.

3. Pour the smoothie into 2 glasses and serve immediately.

Serves 2.

Peachy Coconut Juice

Calories: 190 per serving (½ of recipe)

Coconut water is an excellent liquid to include in your detox diet. Not only does it help to keep your body hydrated, but it also helps improve circulation, which will enhance your blood's ability to filter toxins.

- 3 cups frozen peaches
- 2 cups coconut water
- 1 frozen banana
- 1 teaspoon vanilla extract
- Pinch of salt

---

1. Combine all of the ingredients in a blender. Blend the mixture until smooth.

2. Pour into 2 glasses and serve immediately.

Serves 2.

Garden Green Juice with Nori

Calories: 100 per serving (½ of recipe)

Green vegetables are excellent for detoxing the body because they contain a variety of vitamins and minerals. Many vegetables also contain substances that help increase bile production and liver function to flush toxins out of your system.

- 1 cup baby spinach leaves
- 1 cup chopped kale leaves
- 1 small cucumber, quartered
- 1 large stalk celery

- 5 sprigs fresh parsley
- 5 sprigs fresh cilantro
- 1 medium pear, halved
- 1 tablespoon dried nori flakes

---

1. Feed all the ingredients except the nori through a juicer according to the manufacturer's instructions.

2. Stir the dried nori flakes into the juice.

3. Pour the juice into 2 glasses and serve immediately.

Serves 2.

Berry Flaxseed Smoothie

Calories: 160 per serving (½ of recipe)

This smoothie is sweet and flavorful, which makes it a great option for a healthful dessert. As an alternative, try this delicious smoothie for breakfast.

- 1 cup frozen strawberries
- 1 cup frozen blueberries
- 1 cup frozen raspberries
- 1 cup orange juice
- 2 tablespoons ground flaxseed
- 1 tablespoon raw honey (optional)

1. Combine the berries in a blender and pulse to chop. Add the orange juice and blend the mixture until smooth. Add the remaining ingredients and blend until smooth.

2. Pour the smoothie into 2 glasses and serve immediately.

Serves 2.

Cucumber Kale Juice

Calories: 160 per recipe

This cucumber kale juice is easy to make and full of nutrients. In addition to meeting almost half your daily recommendation for fruits and vegetables, this juice is loaded with potassium, vitamin B, and vitamin C.

- ½ lemon or lime
- 1 English cucumber, cut into 1-inch chunks
- 2 large kale leaves, trimmed
- 1 medium apple, cored

1. Feed the lemon or lime through the juicer, followed by about half of the cucumber chunks.

2. Add the kale leaves next, followed by the apple and the remaining cucumber.

3. Pour the juice into a glass and serve immediately.

Serves 1.

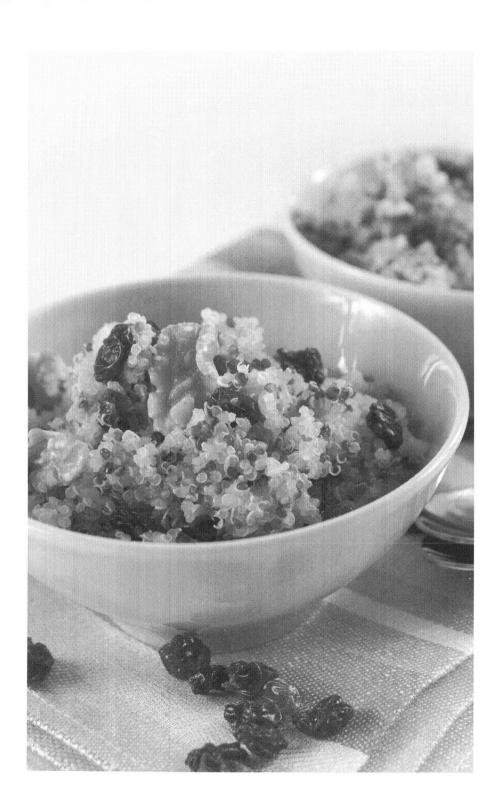

11

BEAUTIFUL SNACKS AND ENERGY BOOSTERS

If you are engaging in a detox diet with the goal of losing weight in mind, it is important to divide your daily calories correctly. Rather than eating most of your daily calories in one meal, try to space them evenly throughout the day. Eat three light or moderate meals alternately with healthful snacks. The snacks in this section are full of detoxifying ingredients that will help you achieve success on your detox diet.

Coconut-Stuffed Dates

Calories: 75 per date

These coconut-stuffed dates are a unique snack that are sure to satisfy your cravings. Made with naturally sweet pitted dates and coconut, they will definitely take your taste buds for a ride.

- ¾ cup young coconut meat
- ½ cup unsweetened coconut milk
- ½ cup raw honey
- ½ cup unsweetened coconut
- 2 tablespoons coconut oil
- Pinch of salt
- 24 pitted Medjool dates

1. Combine all the ingredients except the dates in a blender. Blend the mixture until smooth and well combined.

2. Spoon about 1 tablespoon of the mixture into each date and arrange on a plate.

3. Top with extra coconut, if desired, and chill for 15 minutes before serving.

Makes 24 stuffed dates.

No-Bake Raisin Date Balls

Calories: 130 per ball

If you are looking for a snack that is easy to take on the go, these no-bake raisin date balls are the perfect choice. It takes only a few minutes to whip up a batch, and you can toss them in a plastic bag and take them wherever you go.

- 1 cup chopped pitted dates
- 1 cup raisins
- ½ cup chopped walnuts
- 1 cup raw cashews
- ½ teaspoon vanilla extract
- Pinch of salt

---

1. Combine the dates and raisins in a food processor and pulse until finely chopped.

2. Transfer the dried fruit to a mixing bowl.

3. Place the walnuts and cashews in the food processor and pulse to chop.

4. Add the nuts to the dried fruit and stir in the vanilla extract and salt.

5. Knead the mixture by hand and shape it into 1-inch balls.

6. Chill the balls until ready to serve.

Makes about 20 balls.

Pink Grapefruit Sorbet

Calories: 120 per ½-cup serving

Citrus fruits such as grapefruit are full of the natural sugars your body needs for energy. They are also packed with vitamins and minerals that will restore your body to its natural function.

- 3 pink grapefruit, peeled
- 3 cups water
- 1 cup raw honey
- 1 ripe frozen banana
- 1 tablespoon fresh lemon juice

1. Using a small, sharp knife, carefully separate the grapefruit's pulp from the membranes.

2. Combine all of the ingredients in a food processor or blender and blend until smooth and well combined.

3. Pour the ingredients into an ice-cream maker and freeze according to the manufacturer's instructions.

Serves 2.

Cinnamon Baked-Apple Chips

Calories: 85 per 1-cup serving

These are an excellent alternative to potato chips. They will satisfy your need for a crunchy snack while providing you with all of the nutritional benefits of apples.

- 4 medium apples, cored
- 1 tablespoon ground cinnamon

- 2 teaspoons raw honey (optional)

---

1. Preheat oven to 325 degrees F and line a baking sheet with parchment paper.

2. Slice the apples as thinly as possible and spread them on the baking sheet.

3. Sprinkle the slices with cinnamon and drizzle with honey.

4. Bake the apples for 30 minutes and then carefully flip them with a spatula.

5. Bake the apples for another 40–50 minutes until they are dried.

6. Turn off the oven and let the apples sit until they are crisp.

Serves 4.

Cherry Oatmeal Bars

Calories: 200 per bar

Whether you are in the mood for a tasty snack or you are looking for a quick, grab-and-go breakfast, these cherry oatmeal bars will hit the spot.

- Cooking oil for greasing
- 2 cups old-fashioned oats
- 2 teaspoons ground cinnamon
- 1½ teaspoons baking powder
- ¼ teaspoon salt
- 1 cup unsweetened almond milk
- ½ cup unsweetened applesauce
- 1 large egg
- ¼ cup raw honey
- 1 teaspoon almond extract
- ½ cup chopped dried cherries

1. Preheat oven to 350 degrees F and lightly grease an 8 x 8–inch baking pan with cooking oil.

2. Whisk together the oats, cinnamon, baking powder, and salt in a mixing bowl.

3. Stir in the almond milk and applesauce and then beat in the egg.

4. Whisk in the honey and almond extract until the mixture is smooth and then fold in the chopped cherries.

5. Pour the mixture into the prepared pan and bake for 30–35 minutes until the bars are set and lightly browned.

6. Cool the mixture completely before cutting into bars.

Makes 8 bars.

Toasted Coconut Trail Mix

Calories: 260 per ⅓-cup serving

This toasted coconut trail mix is the ultimate detox snack. Not only is it full of fiber, protein, and antioxidants but it is also portable.

- ½ cup toasted pine nuts
- ½ cup toasted almonds
- ½ cup raisins
- ¼ cup toasted walnuts
- ¼ cup dried cranberries
- ¼ cup toasted coconut

1. Combine all of the ingredients in a mixing bowl and stir until well combined.

2. Transfer the trail mix to an airtight container and store up to 1 week.

Makes about 2¼ cups.

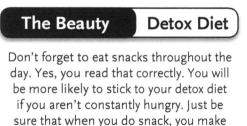

The Beauty Detox Diet

Don't forget to eat snacks throughout the day. Yes, you read that correctly. You will be more likely to stick to your detox diet if you aren't constantly hungry. Just be sure that when you do snack, you make healthful choices.

Raw Sesame Fruit Balls

Calories: 150 per ball

Healthful food doesn't have to be bland and boring. These raw sesame fruit balls are proof that food that is good for you can look good, too. Try these snacks out at your next dinner party and you may be surprised by all of the compliments you receive.

- 1 cup chopped pitted dates
- ½ cup dried cranberries
- ½ cup raisins
- 1 cup raw cashews
- ½ teaspoon vanilla extract
- Pinch of salt
- ¼ cup raw sesame seeds

1. Combine the dates, cranberries, and raisins in a food processor and pulse until finely chopped.

2. Add the cashews, vanilla extract, and salt and pulse until the mixture begins to stick together in a ball.

3. Turn the mixture out onto a sheet of waxed paper and knead by hand, shaping into 1-inch balls.

4. Roll the balls in the raw sesame seeds to coat them and then arrange them on a plate.

5. Chill the balls until ready to serve.

Makes about 20 balls.

Orange Raspberry Sherbet

Calories: 130 per ½-cup serving

The perfect combination of fresh fruit flavors, this orange raspberry sherbet is refreshing and full of valuable nutrients. This treat is the perfect snack to enjoy during your detox.

- 1½ cups cold unsweetened almond milk
- 1 cup orange juice
- 1 cup frozen raspberries
- ¾ cup raw honey
- 2 tablespoons orange zest
- 1 tablespoon fresh lemon juice

1. Combine all of the ingredients in a food processor or blender, and blend until smooth and well combined.

2. Pour the mixture into an ice-cream maker and freeze according to the manufacturer's instructions.

Serves 8.

Agave Sunflower Granola Bars

Calories: 220 per bar

These granola bars are like nothing you will find at the supermarket. Made with healthful oats, nuts, and seeds, these bars have all the fiber and protein you need to tide you over until your next meal.

- Cooking oil for greasing
- 1 cup old-fashioned oats
- 1 cup chopped walnuts
- ½ cup raw sunflower seeds
- ½ cup sifted coconut flour
- ½ cup raisins
- ¼ cup coconut oil, meltedl
- 2 teaspoons almond extract
- Pinch of salt
- ½ cup agave nectar

1. Lightly grease a rectangular glass baking dish with cooking oil.

2. Place the oats, walnuts, and sunflower seeds in a food processor and pulse until finely chopped.

3. Pour the mixture into a bowl and stir in the coconut flour. Add the raisins, coconut oil, almond extract, and salt and then stir until the mixture is well combined.

4. Heat the agave in the microwave for 5–10 seconds and then pour it into the mixing bowl.

5. Stir the mixture well and then transfer it to the glass baking dish.

6. Spread the mixture evenly and then chill until firm. Cut into bars to serve.

Makes 12 bars.

Roasted Curry Cauliflower Bites

Calories: 120 per 1-cup serving

These bites are the ultimate healthful snack for a detox diet. Cauliflower contains glucosinolates, which help boost and regulate your body's detoxification enzymes.

- 1 head cauliflower
- 2 tablespoons olive oil
- 1 teaspoon curry powder
- Pinch of salt
- Red pepper flakes, as desired

---

1. Preheat oven to 425 degrees F.

2. Chop the cauliflower into bite-sized florets, and spread them on a rimmed baking sheet.

3. Drizzle the cauliflower with the oil and sprinkle with curry powder and salt.

4. Roast for 20 minutes, stirring occasionally, until the cauliflower just begins to brown.

5. Sprinkle the cauliflower with red pepper flakes, if desired, and serve warm.

Serves 4.

Raw Chocolate Truffles

Calories: 85 per truffle

These delicious chocolate truffles will have you reconsidering the notion that healthful food can't be tasty.

- 1½ cups cashews
- 2 cups water
- ¾ cup unsweetened cocoa
- ⅔ cup raw honey
- 1 teaspoon almond extract
- ½ teaspoon ground cinnamon
- ½ teaspoon salt
- ¾ cup cocoa butter

1. Soak the cashews in the water for 2–4 hours and then drain.

2. Combine the cashews, cocoa, honey, almond extract, cinnamon, salt, and cocoa butter in a food processor and mix until smooth.

3. Spoon the mixture into a bowl and chill for 20 minutes or until firm enough to mold by hand.

4. Shape the mixture into 1-inch balls.

5. Place the truffles on a plate and serve immediately.

Serves 4.

Sesame Kale Chips

Calories: 125 per 1-cup serving

Kale is sometimes called a super food because it contains a wealth of healthful nutrients. When kale is chewed, it produces a substance called sulforaphane, which helps your liver produce detoxifying enzymes.

- 2 bunches kale
- ¼ cup olive oil
- 1 tablespoon fresh lemon juice
- ½ cup raw sesame seeds
- Pinch of salt

---

1. Preheat oven to 200 degrees F and line a baking sheet with parchment paper.

2. Rinse the kale and remove the stems. Chop the leaves into 2-inch chunks.

3. Place the kale in a bowl and drizzle with olive oil and lemon juice.

4. Toss the kale with the sesame seeds and salt until coated and then spread on the baking sheet.

5. Bake for 30 minutes and then flip the kale with a spatula.

6. Bake for another 20 minutes or so until the kale is dried and crispy.

7. Cool the kale chips completely before serving.

Serves 4.

Coconut Cashew Date Bars

Calories: 180 per bar

For a quick energy boost, these coconut cashew date bars will do the trick. Loaded with dietary fiber and protein, these snacks are sure to keep you going.

- 2 cups chopped pitted dates
- 1½ cups raw cashews
- ¼ cup unsweetened flaked coconut
- ½ teaspoon coconut extract
- Pinch of salt

1. Combine all of the ingredients in a food processor and pulse to chop. Blend the ingredients until they begin to stick together and form a ball. (This could take several minutes.)

2. Transfer the mixture to a glass baking dish and spread it evenly with your fingers.

3. Chill the mixture until set, about 20 minutes, and then cut into bars to serve.

Makes about 6 bars.

Cinnamon Chia Pudding

Calories: 240 per ½-cup serving

Chia seeds are rich in both soluble and insoluble fiber, which helps to clean out your digestive tract. These seeds will also enhance your body's ability to absorb fat-soluble vitamins like A, C, and E.

- ⅔ cup chia seeds
- 2 cups unsweetened almond milk
- 2 teaspoons ground cinnamon
- 1 teaspoon almond extract
- Pinch of salt
- Fresh fruit (optional)

---

1. Place the chia seeds in a medium bowl.

2. Whisk together the remaining ingredients except the fruit in a separate bowl, and pour the mixture over the chia seeds.

3. Stir the mixture well, cover, and let sit for 2 hours or until the chia seeds absorb the moisture, forming a tapioca-like consistency.

4. Serve the pudding with fresh fruit, if desired.

Serves 2.

Raisin-Stuffed Baked Apples

Calories: 120 per apple

These baked apples are warm and tender, the perfect treat for a snack or dessert. Best of all? It's good for you.

- Cooking oil for greasing
- 4 medium apples, cored
- ¼ cup unsweetened shredded coconut
- ¼ cup raisins
- 2 tablespoons coconut oil
- 1 teaspoon ground cinnamon
- Pinch ground nutmeg

1. Preheat oven to 350 degrees F and lightly grease a glass baking dish with cooking oil.

2. Arrange the apples in the baking dish and set aside.

3. Combine the remaining ingredients in a bowl and stir well.

4. Stuff the raisin mixture into the apples and then bake for 40 minutes until tender.

Serves 4.

CONCLUSION

After reading this book, you may find yourself facing some difficult truths. You may be realizing that your diet is a lot less healthful than you thought it was. Or perhaps you now fully understand the dangers of commercial beauty products and environmental toxins. Don't feel ashamed if this is the first time you have really thought about these things—the fact that you are thinking them now means that you are ready to begin your detox.

Not only are you equipped with the knowledge of what kind of benefits a detox has in store for you, but you also understand *why* it works and *how*. The detox is not just another slim-quick scheme—it isn't even centered on the goal of losing weight. The goal of the detox diet is to cleanse your body of the toxins that are holding you back, freeing you to achieve your full potential.

In following the guidelines of the detox diet, you will find that you feel more vital and energized than you have in a long time. Your skin will be smooth and clear, your hair sleek and shiny, your nails strong and healthy. All of these benefits and more are within your reach. All you have to do is take the first step. Eliminate the foods and products that introduce toxins into your body and replace them with naturally detoxifying foods. The recipes included in this book will help you get started with the detox diet, and once you get started, you will never want to stop. Good luck and thanks for reading.

GLOSSARY

adipose tissue—the type of tissue used by the body to store energy in the form of lipids (fat); typically found beneath the skin, but in cases where there is too much adipose tissue, it can begin to back up in and around the organs.

aflatoxin—a mycotoxin produced by the type of mold often found in peanuts; one of the most carcinogenic substances known to man.

age-related disease—a disease occurring most frequently or with increasing frequency among older individuals; also, a disease or complication resulting from an individual's advancement in age.

aging process—the natural process through which bodily cells die and regenerate. The process begins with birth and the rate of cell death increases with age.

artificial sweetener—synthetic sweeteners (not derived from natural sugars) such as aspartame, saccharin, sucralose, and sugar alcohols.

biotoxins—toxins produced by microorganisms.

bisphenol A (BPA)—a type of chemical used to line soda cans; it has been linked to birth defects and improper development in children.

cleanse—to remove impurities or to wash clean.

colon hydrotherapy—also known as a colonic, this is a procedure used to cleanse the colon by injecting water into the colon through the rectum.

cynarin—a naturally occurring chemical that increases bile production and liver function.

detox—the removal of a harmful substance, such as a poison or toxin; also, this refers to the act of following a particular diet or engaging in certain eating habits in order to cleanse the body of accumulated toxins.

enzymes—molecules responsible for catalyzing bodily processes.

exorphins—substances produced by the body in response to opioids (peptides found in grains) that increase appetite and food cravings.

fast—the act of abstaining from food, liquid, or both for a defined period of time.

galactose—a simple sugar found in dairy products and some other foods that has been linked to ovarian cancer and inhibited immune function.

gluten—a protein found in wheat, barley, and rye.

goitrogens—a type of compound that suppresses the healthy function of the thyroid gland.

lectins—carbohydrate-binding proteins, which can be very toxic to the human body if consumed in excess or not properly cooked.

mycotoxin—a toxic substance produced by mold.

neurotransmitters—the chemicals found in the brain that transmit signals, facilitating communication between brain and nerve cells.

phthalates—chemical compounds containing phthalic acid, which are found in many types of plastics, including water bottles, food containers, and toys.

phytates—substances found in grains and soy that bind to certain minerals such as calcium, iron, magnesium, and zinc, making your body unable to absorb those nutrients.

preservatives—substances added to food to prevent spoiling or to increase the shelf life of a product.

probiotics—bacteria that help promote healthy digestion by encouraging balance in the microflora of the intestines; the word probiotic may also be applied to dietary supplements containing live bacteria taken for the purpose of improving gut health and digestion.

refining—the process through which foods (such as sugar or flour) are altered to isolate the starch. This process often results in a loss of over 50 percent of the nutritional value of the food.

selenium—a trace element found in many foods that plays a critical role in reproduction, thyroid hormone metabolism, and white blood cell production.

small intestinal bacterial overgrowth (SIBO)—a condition in which the bacteria in the small intestine reproduce too rapidly.

toxin—a harmful substance that can cause serious health problems, even in small doses.

REFERENCES AND RESOURCES

AARC (Alzheimer's and Aging Research Center). "Common Age Related Diseases." AARC. http://www.aging-research.org/diseases.html. (Accessed June 5, 2013.)

Arculeo, Steven. "Toxins—The Surprising Reason for Weight Gain." Chicago Healers. April 1, 2009. http://www.chicagohealers.com/press-releases/pr1-apr09/.

Bunch, Kimberly. "Release Toxins from the Body Naturally." Yahoo! Voices. June 9, 2009. http://voices.yahoo.com/release-toxins-body-naturally-3446072.html?cat=5.

CDC (Center on the Developing Child). "Toxic Stress: The Facts." CDC at Harvard University. http://developingchild.harvard.edu/topics/science_of_early_childhood/toxic_stress_response/. (Accessed June 5, 2013.)

CHEJ (Center for Health, Environment and Justice). "Frequently Asked Questions about Dioxin and Food." CHEJ. January 30, 2012. http://chej.org/wp-content/uploads/Frequently-Asked-Questions-About-Dioxin-and-Food.pdf.

Children's Environmental Health Project. "Dermatological Effects." Canadian Association of Physicians for the Environment. http://www.cape.ca/children/derm.html. (Accessed June 5, 2013.)

Cornell College. "What Processes Does the Liver Undergo to Remove Toxins?" Cornell College. http://people.cornellcollege.edu/bnowakthompson/pdfs/liverDetox.pdf. (Accessed June 5, 2013.)

Danna, Jim, and Jo Jordan. "Glazed and Confused. It's Time to Wake Up and Smell the Coffee." Puristat. http://www.puristat.com/standardamericandiet/processedfoods.aspx. (Accessed June 7, 2013.)

Merriam-Webster Online. s.v. "detoxify." http://www.merriam-webster.com/dictionary/detoxification. (Accessed June 6, 2013.)

Dickinson, Dave. "Top 10 Most Dangerous Environmental Toxins in the U.S." Listosaur.com. September 6, 2011. http://listosaur.com/science-a-technology/top-10-most-dangerous-environmental-toxins-in-the-u.s.html.

Ewers, Keela. "Where Do Toxins Come From: 'Detoxification . . . Restore Your Core'" Natural Choice Directory. http://www.naturalchoice.net/articles/Art11_Toxins.htm. (Accessed June 5, 2013.)

Foster, Daniel W. 1967. "Studies in the Ketosis of Fasting." *Journal of Clinical Investigation* 46 (8): 1283–96. doi:10.1172/JCI105621.

Group, Edward F. "Daily Toxin Intake." Global Healing Center. http://www.globalhealingcenter.com/health-hazards-to-know-about/daily-toxin-intake. (Accessed June 7, 2013.)

Hamid, Rabia, and Akbar Masood. 2009. "Dietary Lectins as Disease Causing Intoxicants." *Pakistan Journal of Nutrition* 8 (3): 293–303. http://www.pjbs.org/pjnonline/fin1120.pdf

Hines, Elisabeth. "Toxins and Toxic Overload." Health by Design. http://www.mybodycanhealitself.ca/toxins_and_toxic_overload.htm. (Accessed June 7, 2013.)

Hyman, Mark. "Is There Toxic Waste in Your Body?" Dr. Hyman. May 19, 2010. http://drhyman.com/blog/2010/05/19/ is-there-toxic-waste-in-your-body-2/#close.

Katie. "Why You Should Never Eat Vegetable Oil or Margarine." Wellness Mama. http://wellnessmama.com/2193/why-you-should-never-eat-vegetable-oil-or-margarine/. (Accessed June 6, 2013.)

Lanou, Amy Joy, Susan E. Berkow, and Neal D. Barnard. 2005. "Calcium, Dairy Products, and Bone Health in Children and Young Adults: A Reevaluation of the Evidence." *Pediatrics: Official Journal of the American Academy of Pediatrics* 115 (3): 736–43. http://pediatrics.aappublications.org/content/115/3/736.abstract.

Lin, Julie, and Gary C. Curhan. 2011. "Associations of Sugar and Artificially Sweetened Soda with Albuminuria and Kidney Function Decline in Women." *Clinical Journal of the American Society of Nephrology* 6 (1): 160–6. doi: 10.2215/CJN.03260410.

Lipik, Vitaly. "Dioxin Becomes Most Dangerous Man-Made Poison." Pravda.ru. January 6, 2005. http://english.pravda.ru/science/ tech/01-06-2005/8345-dioxin-0/.

LivLong Inc. "The Liver's Crucial Role in Weight Loss." http:// livlong.ca/374/the-livers-crucial-role-in-weight-loss. (Accessed June 5, 2013.)

Murray, Joseph A. 1999. "The Widening Spectrum of Celiac Disease." *American Journal of Clinical Nutrition* 69 (3): 354–65. http://ajcn. nutrition.org/content/69/3/354.full.

NRDC (Natural Resources Defense Council). "Environment and Health." NRDC. http://www.nrdc.org/health/. (Accessed June 7, 2013.)

Paleo Diet Lifestyle. "The Dangers of Soy." http://paleodietlifestyle. com/dangers-soy/. (Accessed June 5, 2013.)

Perkins, Cynthia. "Get Rid of Adult Acne from the Inside Out." *Holistic Health Talk* (blog). August 7, 2008. http://www.holis- tichelp.net/blog/get-rid-of-acne-from-the-inside-out/.

Redwin, Breanna. "How to Get Clear Skin with a Detox Cleanse." Suite 101. December 15, 2009. http://suite101.com/article/ how-to-get-clear-skin-with-a-detox-cleanse-a180314.

Remove Body Toxins. "Understanding Antiaging . . . You Must Understand Aging." http://www.remove-body-toxins.com/ antiaging.html. (Accessed June 5, 2013.)

Richards, Byron J. "Unclog Your Liver and Lose Abdominal Fat— Leptin Diet Weight Loss Challenge #6." Wellness Resources. May 7, 2012. http://www.wellnessresources.com/weight/articles/ unclog_your_liver_lose_your_abdominal_fat_leptin_diet_ weight_loss_challenge/.

Scarlata, Kate. 2011. "Small Intestinal Bacterial Overgrowth—What to Do When Unwelcome Microbes Invade." *Today's Dietician* 13 (4): 46. http://www.todaysdietitian.com/newarchives/040511p46. shtml.

Sinclair, Janelle. "How Exposure to Toxins Can Cause Depression, Anxiety and Other Mental Health Illnesses." *Breaking Free from Depression* (blog). http://www.breakingfreefromdepression.com/ exposure-to-toxins-can-cause-depression-anxiety/. (Accessed June 7, 2013.)

Sinha, Rashmi, Amanda J. Cross, Barry I. Graubard, Michael F. Leitzmann, and Arthur Schatzkin. 2009. "Meat Intake and Mortality: A Prospective Study of Over Half a Million People." *Archives of Internal Medicine* 169 (6): 562–71. http://www.ncbi. nlm.nih.gov/pubmed/19307518.

Why Detox. "How to Start Detoxing." *Detox Blog.* http://whydetox. net/how-to-start-detoxing. (Accessed June 6, 2013.)

Why Detox. "Skin Detoxification." *Detox Blog.* http://whydetox.net/ skin-detoxification. (Accessed June 6, 2013.)

Zelman, Kathleen M. "The Truth about Detox Diets." WebMD. http:// www.webmd.com/food-recipes/guide/detox-diets-purging-myths. (Accessed June 6, 2013.)

INDEX

Made in the USA
Lexington, KY
22 January 2014